KU-285-124

Diagnosis in color

Sexually Transmitted Diseases

Second Edition

Anthony Wisdom
MB, BS (London)
Consultant Physician
Oldchurch and Newham Hospitals
London
UK

David A Hawkins
BSc, FRCP
Consultant Physician
St Stephen's Centre
Chelsea and Westminster Hospital
London
UK

M Mosby-Wolfe
MEDICAL COMMUNICATIONS

Development Editor:	**Gina Almond**
Project Manager:	**Peter Harrison**
Production:	**Hamish Adamson**
Index:	**Anita Reid**
Design:	**Greg Smith**
Layout:	**Rob Curran**
Illustrators:	**Lynda Payne/John Cheung**
Cover Design:	**Gisli Thor**
Publisher:	**Rebecca Whitehead**

MOSBY
An imprint of Harcourt Publishers Limited

M is a registered trademark of Harcourt Publishers Limited

© Mosby-Wolfe 1997
© Harcourt Publishers Limited 1999

First published in 1997 by Mosby-Wolfe
  Reprinted 1999
ISBN 0 7234 2496 9

British Library Cataloguing in Publication Data
A catalogue record for this book is available from the British Library.

Printed in Spain by Elkar S. Coop

Contents

Preface to the Second Edition

Patterns in all fields of modern medicine are changing at an accelerating rate. This is mainly due to the many advances in knowledge of pathogenesis and, specifically in the field of communicable disease, to increased understanding of microorganisms, with consequent improvement in diagnosis and therapy. The specialty of genitourinary medicine is particularly involved because of the many millions of individuals affected, directly and indirectly, by the human immunodeficiency virus (HIV). Thus the time has come for a further revision of this established book and I am fortunate to have been joined by Dr David Hawkins of the Chelsea and Westminster Hospital as co-author.

We have completely revised the first edition to encompass advances in diagnostic techniques and in the knowledge of disease processes. The 'old' venereal diseases of syphilis (particularly in its late stages and congenital disease) and gonorrhoea have considerably declined in frequency in industrialized countries, though vigilance is still required to keep these traditional STDs under control—for example, a decrease in routine antenatal clinic testing contributed to the outbreak of early infectious and congenital syphilis in central New York in the 1980s. Conversely, chlamydial infections and non-specific genital infections in general and their complications appear to be much more numerous, partly because of the wider availability of non-cultural diagnostic tests.

Transmission of infectious agents by sexual contact is now recognized in an increasing number of diseases (well beyond the number of statutorily defined conditions in the UK) and the complexity of these, often multisystem, disorders is better understood. For example, the genital manifestations of herpes simplex infections may cause much morbidity, both physical and psychological. There is also more understanding of the role of human papilloma virus (HPV) in cervical neoplasia and marked concern about the long-term effect on reproductive health of chlamydial and other genital tract infections. In underdeveloped countries with poor resources for health care, the traditional venereal diseases are still extremely common, with the medical problems being compounded by poverty, malnutrition and urbanization with a poor infrastructure (and lack of emancipation for women!). Infection with HIV now affects an estimated 20 million people worldwide, with most infections acquired through heterosexual activity. Inevitably, there are already tragically large numbers of children affected by HIV, either by vertical transmission or by becoming orphans of parents who have died of this disease. The socioeconomic consequences are incalculable, but obviously profound.

HIV infection has focused the attention of many talented researchers in diverse fields. The work of these researchers is also yielding new knowledge of other sexually transmitted diseases and on human sexual behaviour. HIV infection may directly affect the clinical course of the older sexually transmitted diseases. Understanding such interactions is important and is particularly emphasized in the text.

As we have previously emphasized, the role of health education (for the general public) is absolutely crucial in the arena of genital problems. The only way that an individual will change from 'risk' to 'safe' patterns of behaviour is through knowledge and understanding of what is 'risky' and what is 'safe'. This has been underlined particularly by the public reaction to HIV disease, in which groups of laypeople have taken on a most important role in providing advice and information, often targeted to specific groups, such as homosexuals, young people and immigrants. These voluntary bodies also often provide advice and information in areas where conventional allopathic medicine does not venture. Finally, I (ARW) would like again to repeat the last words of the preface to previous editions: '....treatment....must include sympathetic understanding and reassurance of the patient who is so often acutely anxious about his or her condition'. Thirty years on, this is still very true.

Anthony Wisdom
David Hawkins
London 1997

Acknowledgements to the Second Edition

The majority of the new illustrations in the current edition were taken by staff of the Medical Illustration Department of the Chelsea & Westminster Hospital or from its former incarnation on the same site at St Stephen's Hospital and also at the former Westminster Hospital. We would like to thank them for their enthusiasm and for the quality of the pictures achieved, which are a credit to their expertise.

David Hawkins would like to thank his colleagues in the HIV/GUM directorate at the Chelsea & Westminster Hospital, in particular Dr Adam Lawrence, who read through an early draft and provided many pictures for both the current, as well as the previous, edition. Other consultant colleagues who have generously donated slides from their collections include: Dr Brian Gazzard; Dr Simon Barton; Dr Fiona Boag; Dr Mark Nelson and Dr Priya Samrasinghe. Further material was provided by Dr Barbara Vonau, Dr Dan Sharpstone, Dr Mike Youle, Dr Graeme Moyle, Dr Michael Connolly, Dr John Keating and Jenny Midgely. We are fortunate to have had close links with our dermatologists, in particular Dr Richard Staughton and Dr Chris Bunker, both of whom provided many illustrations and gave much help and advice on skin conditions—both HIV and non-HIV alike. Other significant contributions were from Dr Nick Francis, who provided the histopathology slides, Dr Jerry Healey, who contributed to and reviewed the radiology images; Dr Suzanne Mitchell (Ophthalmology section) and Drs Martin Brueton and Jennifer Evans (Paediatrics),

Dr Roberto Guilloff (Neurology), Dr Christine Costello (Haematology) and Dr Bob Phillips (Radiotherapy and Oncology).

Other than our local colleagues, we would also like to thank Professors David Taylor-Robinson, Jonathan Weber, Anthony Pinching and Dr Willy Harris (all currently or formerly at St Mary's Hospital, Paddington); Dr Phillip Hay at St George's Hospital, Dr Diane Bennett at the PHLS Colindale, Professor Gerry Stimson at the Centre for Research on Drugs and Health Behaviour, Charing Cross and Westminster Medical School and Professor David Mabey, London School of Hygiene and Tropical Medicine.

Finally, we would like to thank all at Mosby International, including Richard Furn, Gina Almond and Peter Harrison for encouragement and for maintaining the momentum of the project. A number of secretarial staff have been of great help, including Robyn Holmes and Carlene Givans-Grant.

Anthony Wisdom
David Hawkins
London 1997

Preface to the First Edition

Since the first version of this book was published, under the title of *A Colour Atlas of Venereology,* there have been many changes, some minor and some major. Even the accepted title of the specialty has changed to **genitourinary medicine** partly to diminish the pejorative associations of the former title, **venereology**, but also to reflect the changing patterns of morbidity of relevant conditions within the community.

In this edition I have added a section on HIV/AIDS which is necessarily brief. Many patients presenting with this condition are first diagnosed in genitourinary medical clinics, and it is likely that much of the subsequent care as outpatients will be managed in these departments. I have considerably changed the section on non-gonococcal infections, mainly because facilities for identification of chlamydial infections are now widespread, allowing more rational management of the condition. New investigative techniques such as colposcopy are included. I have also added many new pictures, both in the new sections and to improve existing ones.

Undoubtedly the major change in genitourinary practice has been the emergence of HIV/AIDS. This severely disabling disease with its high mortality was first recognized in the USA in 1981 and is still too new for the natural history to have been clearly defined, but it is probably the most important medical matter to arise in the second half of the twentieth century. Intially, in developed countries, the disease was found almost exclusively in male homosexuals or the recipients of blood products or transfusions: now it is clear that heterosexual transmission does occur and this is likely to be the main method of spread of infection in the future. At the time of writing no effective therapy is available: treatment at present consists of palliation, both physical and psychological. Of prime importance is the establishment of effective cooperation between health care facilities, social services, local authority services and voluntary organizations in order to help individuals affected by HIV, who have to cope with both their illness and public prejudice. It is already evident that HIV-associated problems can ramify even into the (apparently) most unlikely areas of everyday life.

Two other areas in the specialty also causing concern because of greatly increased frequency of occurrence are covered in this new edition: these are **genital warts** and **pelvic inflammatory disease**. Genital wart (HPV) infections are associated with cervical intraepithelial neoplasia and carcinoma of the cervix, which have been found much more frequently in recent years. especially in younger women. The number of cases of pelvic inflammatory disease has markedly increased, both in genitourinary and gynaecological practice. There has also been an increase in the number of infertile couples who, on investigation, often show signs of previous clinically silent tubal infection in the female, which is known frequently to be caused by sexually transmitted microorganisms. This suggests that we must ensure that screening methods (cervical cytology in HPV, and microbiology in sexually active people not in stable relationships) are freely available and that the public is educated to make use of the resources.

The importance of health education in genitourinary practice has never been in doubt: the recent advent of HIV has emphasized this point. The only practical way at present to reduce transmission of the virus (and other microorganisms) is for individuals to adopt a low-risk lifestyle. My impression is that this message has been received and acted upon by the male homosexual community (as shown by the reduced incidence of sexually transmitted diseases in male homosexuals observed in both the UK and the USA) but there is little evidence as yet that the heterosexual community (particularly those most at risk) have changed their habits.

Finally, I would like to repeat the final words of the introduction to the first version of this book: 'treatment . . . must include sympathetic understanding and reassurance of the patient, who is so often acutely anxious about his or her condition'. All my experience of the past 15 years, and especially since the appearance of HIV, underlines that conclusion.

Anthony Wisdom
London 1989

Acknowledgements to the First Edition

Illustrating this book would have been impossible without the help and kindness of many friends and colleagues who have most generously allowed publication of photographs from their collections. In particular, I thank (and I apologize for any omissions) the following: Dr Suzanne Alexander, Dr June Almeida, Dr J A Armstrong, Dr R D Catterall, Dr G Csonka, Dr E M C Dunlop, Dr A Grimble, Dr J A H Hancock, Dr M J Hare, Mr I A Harper, Dr R N Herson, Dr J J Jefferiss, Mr L Kay, Dr G M Levene, Dr C S Nicol, Dr J K Oates, Dr J D Oriel, Dr G Rohatiner, Mr. H Thomson, Dr D Vollum, Dr A E Wilkinson and Dr R R Willcox; Drs Borchardt and Hoke of San Francisco, Dr Vernal G Cave of New York, Dr W C Duncan of Baylor College, Professor Paolo Nazarro of Rome and Dr T Guthe of WHO, Dr Adam Lawrence, John Hunter Clinic, St Stephen's Hospital, London, who provided the clinical pictures used in the section on HIV disease. Other pictures in this section are taken from *A Colour Atlas of AIDS* (Wolfe), and are published by kind permission of Dr Charles Farthing and his colleagues. Dr A Blackwell for the picture of *Gardnerella vaginalis,* and Dr V R Tindall for illustrations from *A Colour Atlas of Clinical Gynaecology* (Wolfe); the photographic departments of Guy's Hospital, the London Hospital, the Middlesex Hospital, Westminster Hospital, Dr Cardew and the Photographic Department of St Mary's Hospital, Mr E A Shepherd of Oldchurch Hospital, the Trustees of the Wellcome Institute, Messrs May and Baker Ltd and the Venereal Disease Research Unit, Centers for Disease Control, Atlanta, Georgia, USA. I am also very grateful for the constant help given by the nursing staff at my clinics, and for the forbearance and encouragement of the General Editor of the Wolfe Medical Atlases, Dr G Barry Carruthers. I have had much help in preparing the second edition from Maggie King of Mosby-Wolfe Medical Publications, for which I am most grateful.

Anthony Wisdom
London 1989

Dedicated to the staff and colleagues at our clinics who have always been so supportive and helpful, and to the former Association of Technicians in Venereology.

AETIOLOGY OF COMMON PRESENTATIONS

INTRODUCTION

The object of a consultation at a sexual health clinic (sexually transmitted disease (STD) clinic; in the US, STI clinic) is for a conclusion to be made: either the diagnosis or exclusion of disease or disorder. This objective can be achieved only by appraisal of the history, examination and investigation. Patients present for examination either with symptoms of abnormalities of structure or function, or without symptoms when anxious, or as contacts of others already found to have transmissible conditions. Structural abnormalities may be caused by disease or anatomical anomaly: symptoms may be caused by pathological, psychological or physiological processes. Asymptomatic attenders include some without disease but others (including many women and homosexual men) in whom disease can be found only by examination. In this section the evaluation of the history, observed abnormalities and the more common presenting symptoms are outlined, but it is most important to remember that the large group of totally asymptomatic patients require equally careful examination and assessment.

History

Points that should always be noted when taking the history are :

- Current symptoms (if any) and duration. Direct questioning is often helpful.
- Current and recent therapy (prescribed or self-administered).
- Current general health.
- Previous sexually transmitted or other genitourinary disease, general medical history and family history. In patients originating from areas where treponemal disease is endemic, specific enquiry should be made for a history of these conditions.
- Timing of occurrence and type of recent sexual contacts (e.g. marital, casual, homosexual) and any prophylaxis used.
- Presence or absence of genitourinary symptoms in sexual partner.
- (In women) obstetric, gynaecological and menstrual history and contraceptive methods.

The history and examination should always be conducted in a systematic manner: the symptoms and findings will determine further investigations to be undertaken. In the interests of clarity, it is most important that the words and phrases used are understood both by the interviewer and interviewee: medical personnel must always remember that some words and phrases that have a specific connotation to themselves may be used in quite a different sense by patients. Furthermore, many patients will be ignorant of the correct terminology used to describe sexual actions or anatomical parts: it is prudish to refrain from using the vernacular in situations where this would appear to be helpful.

Anatomical anomalies
Variance from the 'normal' is a common reason for attendance, or an anomaly may be found fortuitously. Patients may attend for examination because of a belief that the anomaly, often recently noticed, is a sign of sexually transmitted disease. Recognition is usually straightforward but some conditions, such as phimosis or hypospadias, appear to predispose towards infection and are found more frequently in genitourinary practice than in the general population. The illustrations in this subsection are a selection of anomalies observed in clinical practice.

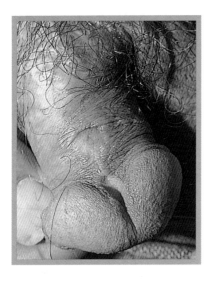

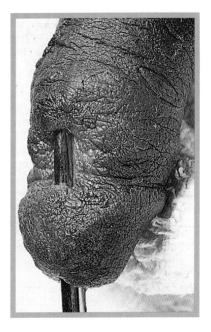

↑ **1 Hypospadias**
The urethral opening is situated on the ventral surface of the penis: the lesion may occur anywhere between the glans and the perineum, and is usually distal. The glans may show a groove in the midline (NB: the penis is rotated in the photograph).

↑ **2 Hypospadias**
The bougie demonstrates the aberrant ventral orifice with canalization of the glans.

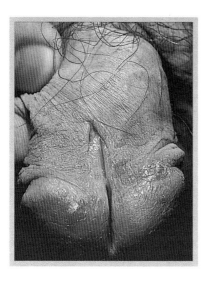

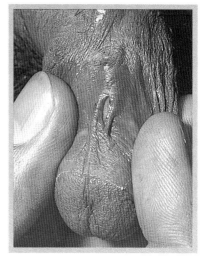

↑ 3 Hypospadias
Note also papular–nodular scabetic lesions.

↑ 4 Median raphe duct
The urethra was normal. The median raphe has remained canalized, causing a short blind sinus.

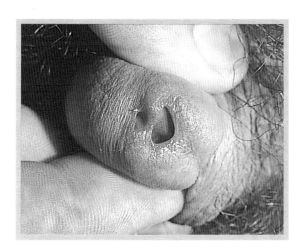

← 5 Para-urethral duct
A common anomaly: usually the duct is shallow and does not communicate with the urethra; rarely, multiple ducts occur.

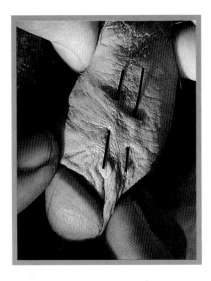

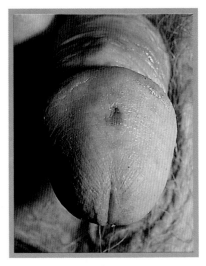

↑ 6 Paired median raphe ducts
A rare anomaly, resulting in this case in the formation of two short tunnels (demonstrated by the bougies).

↑ 7 Dorsal duct
A very rare anomaly (we have never seen another). This patient presented with gonococcal infection of the duct and the urethra and defaulted before investigation of the course of the duct could be undertaken.

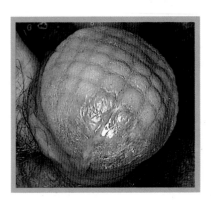

← 8 Oedema of the glans penis
The glans is indented by the pattern of mesh underwear. The patient had non-gonococcal urethritis.

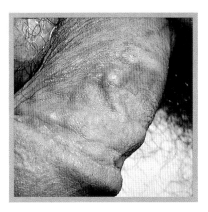

← 9 Lymphocele
Firm translucent thickening of lymph channels proximal to the coronal sulcus. The lesion is caused by blockage of the lymphatics which may follow trauma or infection, but may also occur spontaneously. It is of no significance but may arouse anxiety. In this case the lesion was the sole reason for attendance. This condition is also known as **sclerosing lymphangiitis** or **mucocele**.

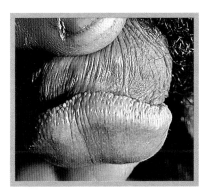

← 10 Pearly penile papules
Physiological fleshy tags on, and adjacent to, the coronal margin, often mistaken for warts.

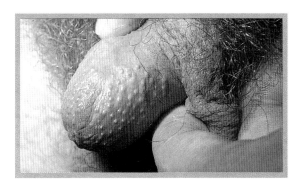

← 11 'Pimples'
A surprisingly frequent reason for attendance by adolescents, who become anxious when such (physiological) small sebaceous glands and hair follicles on the shaft of the penis are first noticed.

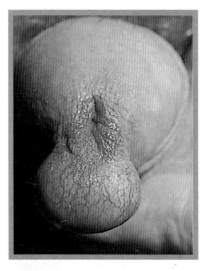

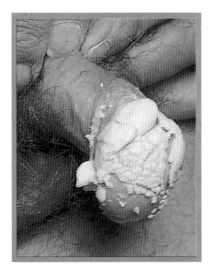

↑ 12 Cyst of frenum
This may require excision or drainage.

↑ 13 Smegma
Lack of hygiene may result in gross accumulation of smegma which may provoke anxiety, or may sometimes cause balanoposthitis.

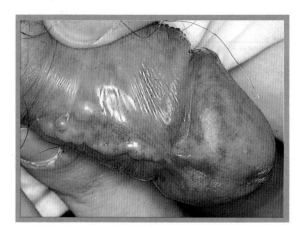

**← 14
Thrombosed
central vein**
Usually post-traumatic. Note also cyst on penile shaft.

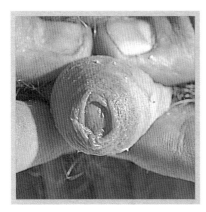

← 15 Preputial adhesion and balanitis
Partial adhesion of the prepuce to the corona has resulted in difficulty in achieving adequate hygiene.

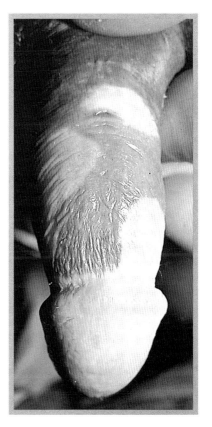

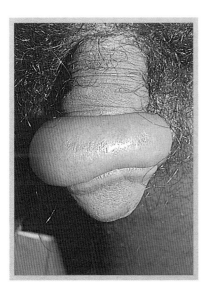

↑ 16 Paraphimosis
The glans has passed through a contracted preputial opening: the contracted band obstructs drainage, causing gross oedema (here confined to the prepuce) distally.

↑ 17 Depigmentation
Postinflammatory, unknown cause. Note rectilinear margins (compare with **18**).

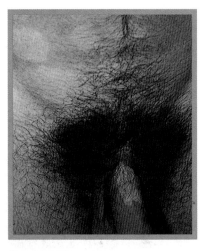

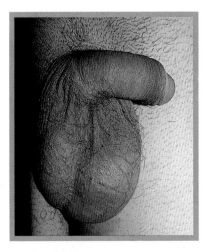

↑ 18 Vitiligo
Note irregular margins (compare with **17**).

↑ 19 Hydrocele
The tense, transilluminable scrotal swelling is usually chronic but occasionally causes attendance in anxious individuals.

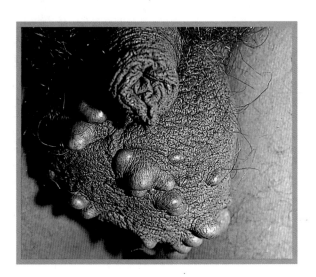

← 20 Multiple sebaceous cysts of the scrotum (steatocystoma multiplex)
Small sebaceous cysts are commonly seen and may become infected: multiple lesions such as these are rare.

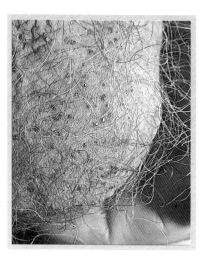

↑ 21 Scrotal angiokeratoma (Fordyce's disease)
These lesions often develop in older people (both male and female).

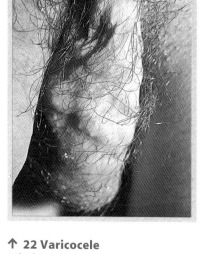

↑ 22 Varicocele
A fairly common reason for attendance in adolescence. The characteristic 'bag of worms' sensation on palpation is diagnostic.

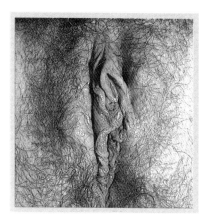

↑ 23 Vulval varix
Often prominent in pregnancy.

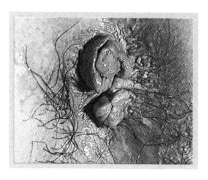

↑ 24 Anal tags
Usually related to piles or a fissure, they may cause anxiety in male homosexuals. A diagnosis of warts may mistakenly be suspected.

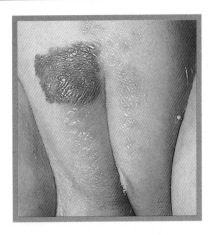

↑ **25 Capillary haemangiomata of vulva.**

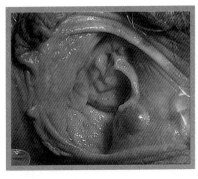

↑ **26 Vulval cyst**
These cysts are usually inclusion cysts following trauma especially during childbirth. Similar cysts occur on the vaginal wall and may result from mesonephric remnants (Gartner's cysts). The cysts are usually noticed fortuitously, but occasionally become infected or cause dyspareunia.

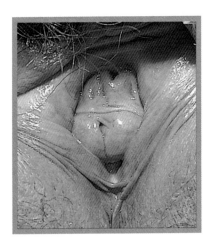

↑ **27 Urethrocele**
Found mainly in older patients.

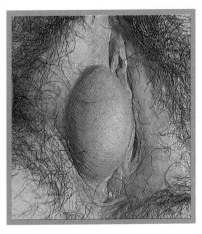

↑ **28 Vulval cyst**
which caused dyspareunia.

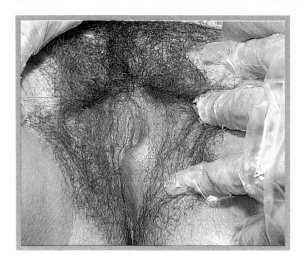

← 29 Bartholin's cyst
Follows duct blockage, partial or complete. Size varies with sexual arousal. Prone to infection.

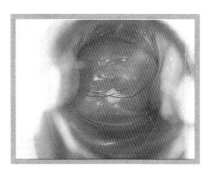

↑ 30 Cervix showing IUCD threads
In practice, the presence of a intrauterine contraceptive device (IUCD) may cause increased vaginal discharge (often bacterial vaginosis, see p. 163) and ascending infection.

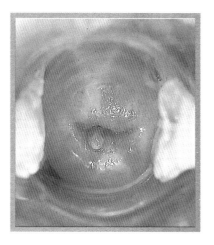

↑ 31 Cervical polyp.

Genital ulcer disease

The presenting complaint is usually an **ulcer** or **sore** which has appeared on or adjacent to the genitalia. Male patients may attend with symptoms of balanoposthitis or preputial oedema: female patients may attend complaining of vulval swelling (oedema): examination reveals underlying ulceration. Ano-receptive homosexuals (and some females) may develop lesions at the anus or on the buttock and upper thigh. Occasionally the initial complaint is of enlarged and/or tender inguinal lymph glands: examination shows active or healed genital ulceration. In some cases lesions on remote parts of the body indicate the need for genital examination which may reveal hitherto unnoticed ulceration. The term **sore** is also used by patients with conditions such as genital warts, herpes, furunculosis or balanoposthitis or it may refer to dysuria or other urinary symptoms.

The importance of a comprehensive history cannot be over-emphasized: some patients are too embarrassed to be truthful on initial attendance and the true history may emerge only when the confidence of the patient has been gained. In conditions such as malignant ulceration, recollection of past deeds may cause the older patient to fear sexually transmitted disease and to consult an STD specialist in the first instance. Any ulcerative lesions should be appropriately investigated, i.e. by dark-field microscopy, bacterial and viral culture, histology or biopsy.

The list of causes shown opposite is not comprehensive: it includes the more frequent and important conditions likely to be encountered in genitourinary practice.

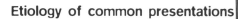

Aetiology of genital ulcer disease		
Group	**Cause**	**Notes**
Infections	Syphilis: primary, secondary, rarely tertiary	
	Lymphogranuloma venereum	Endemic in some tropical and subtropical areas
	Chancroid (soft sore, ulcus molle) Donovanosis }	Principally occurs in tropical areas
	Herpes	Often recurrent. **The most common cause of genital ulceration in North America and Europe**
	Pyogenic	
Trauma	Mechanical damage	May be self-inflicted or caused by injudicious prophylaxis
	Chemical damage	e.g. by phosphonoformate used in treatment of cytomegalovirus (CMV) infections
Neoplastic	Carcinoma Premalignant conditions e.g. erythroplasia of Queyrat; Paget's disease	
Allergic	Fixed drug eruptions	History often diagnostic
	Generalised reactions NB Stevens-Johnson syndrome	
Secondary	In parasitic infestation e.g. scabies, pediculosis	Infestation usually evident at other sites
	Irritant dermatosis	Usually diagnostic evidence elsewhere

↑ **32 Aetiology of genital ulcer disease.**

Lumps in the groin

Lumps in the groin encountered in practice are nearly always of pathological significance, but the cause is often unrelated to sexually transmitted disease or other anogenital conditions. The mass may have been present for some time before attention is sought: conditions such as ectopic location of the testis and hydrocele of the spermatic cord in males, of the canal of Nuck in females and inguinal hernia (direct or indirect) may present in this way. Lesions found below the inguinal ligament that may present in a similar manner include femoral hernia, saphenous varix and arterial aneurysm.

The more significant masses in the groin are caused by **enlargement of the lymphatic glands** (**bubo**), which are normally impalpable, although they may sometimes be detected in thin individuals. Glandular enlargement may be secondary to pyogenic anogenital conditions (often infected parasitic lesions) or to lesions of the leg or abdominal wall: moderate enlargement, often bilateral, and tenderness of the glands is found. Patients with urethritis, balanoposthitis, vulvitis or vaginitis (especially in cases of herpes) are occasionally found to have moderate tender glandular enlargement in association with other symptoms: the glandular symptoms are unlikely to be the presenting feature.

Glandular enlargement is found in about 50% of cases of **primary syphilis**, and may also be found as part of the generalized lymphadenopathy in secondary syphilis. Examination of the syphilitic buboes shows the glands to be firm and rubbery to palpation and moderately enlarged; aggregation and cutaneous involvement does not occur. Moderate tenderness may be experienced but often the enlarged glands are painless.

In **lymphogranuloma venereum** the advent of the bubo is likely to be the first sign of infection, especially in male patients. The bubo may be unilateral or bilateral and is usually painful, irregular and hard, with the glands matted together. Multilocular areas of softening and multiple sinus formation may occur. The skin overlying the bubo is often erythematous and thickened. Characteristically, the glands both above and below the inguinal ligament are involved so that the lesion appears to be traversed by a groove.

In **chancroid** the bubo is similar to that found in lymphogranuloma venereum but the genital primary lesion is usually present. When softening occurs this is unilocular and when a sinus is present this is usually single and associated with adjacent cellulitis.

In **Donovanosis** the mass that is often found in the groin arises from subcutaneous spread of the infection. Abscess and sinus formation may occur: the epithelium adjacent to the sinus shows the characteristic beefy-red granulation tissue.

In **HIV disease** unilateral or bilateral gland enlargement is common; when associated with chronically enlarged glands at other (non-inguinal) locations the condition is known as **persistent generalized lymphadenopathy** (**PGL**). The enlarged glands, usually of moderate size, are discrete; aching discomfort may occur. Enlargement may also occur in seroconversion illness, Kaposi's sarcoma and lymphoma (see pp. 291 and 297).

It is important to remember that enlarged glands may also be caused by conditions such as glandular fever or malignant disease. Reticuloses may first appear in the groin or the glands may be the site of secondary growth from anogenital or remote primary malignant lesions.

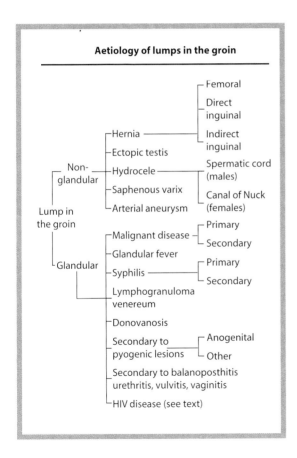

← **33 Aetiology of lumps in the groin.**

23

Anal and perinanal region

Symptoms originating in this area are relatively uncommon in clinical practice but may occur in male anoreceptive homosexuals, some females and, occasionally, in male heterosexuals. Asymptomatic infections are much more frequent.

The commonest symptom is **itching** (**pruritus ani**): it is most important to remember that this symptom is frequently related to stress or anxiety and that patients may associate the complaint with past, guilt-provoking, sexual behaviour. Pruritus ani resulting from organic causes may originate from non-venereal conditions such as haemorrhoids, anal fissure or dermatoses; from venereal conditions such as warts, herpes or other ulceration; or from rectal discharge secondary to conditions such as proctitis or infestation with threadworms or other intestinal parasites e.g. *Giardia lamblia.* Symptomatic candidiasis associated with antibiotic therapy often begins with perianal irritation which may later spread anteriorly. In female patients perianal symptoms may be caused by posterior spread from inflammatory vulval conditions such as candidiasis or trichomoniasis. **Pain** in the anal or perianal region may result from excoriation of irritant lesions or from conditions such as anal fissure; primary herpes simplex of the anus may cause severe pain. Complaint of **rash** in the area may refer to warts or to mycotic or herpetic infection. Tenesmus and constipation are occasionally associated with proctitis, but more commonly with anal fissure or prolapsed piles. **Discharge** from the rectum may be noticed as a sensation of anal dampness or seepage, or the faeces: proctitis is the usual cause. Many female patients with warts on the perineum or at the anus present complaining of 'lumps' in the region, often noticed while washing. Anxious patients with anal tags or prolapse may occasionally consult an STD physician in the first instance.

In **HIV disease**, immunodeficiency may cause severe, painful and persistent recrudescence of ulcerated herpes simplex lesions (see p. 321).

Anal and perianal symptoms

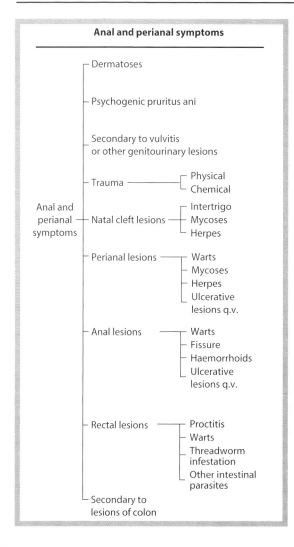

Anal and perianal symptoms
- Dermatoses
- Psychogenic pruritus ani
- Secondary to vulvitis or other genitourinary lesions
- Trauma
  - Physical
  - Chemical
- Natal cleft lesions
  - Intertrigo
  - Mycoses
  - Herpes
- Perianal lesions
  - Warts
  - Mycoses
  - Herpes
  - Ulcerative lesions q.v.
- Anal lesions
  - Warts
  - Fissure
  - Haemorrhoids
  - Ulcerative lesions q.v.
- Rectal lesions
  - Proctitis
  - Warts
  - Threadworm infestation
  - Other intestinal parasites
- Secondary to lesions of colon

← 34 Anal and perianal symptoms.

25

MALE PATIENTS

Most male patients have symptoms and/or abnormal signs at the time of attendance; asymptomatic presentations (anoreceptive homosexuals, contacts or anxious individuals) are less common. In this section the most frequent presenting symptoms (apart from those mentioned previously) are discussed. These symptoms most commonly originate from the prepuce, glans penis and anterior urethra. Less frequently, symptoms may originate from lesions of the scrotum or its contents or more proximal parts of the urinary tract and related structures. The evaluation of genitourinary symptoms in male patients is generally easier than in female patients because the symptoms and their causes are much more likely to be anatomically specific. Lumps in the groin have already been discussed on page 22 and anogenital symptoms on page 24.

Discharge

Complaint of **discharge** usually refers to secretion observed at the end of the penis and is the commonest symptom (but seldom the only one) in practice. Discharge may originate from the urethra or from beneath the prepuce: rarely, the origin may be from another orifice, such as Tyson's gland or a median raphe duct. Discharge may result from physiological causes (e.g. prostatorrhoea, nocturnal emission), local pathological causes (e.g. balanoposthitis, urethritis, trauma) or to lesions of the upper urinary tract: sometimes the symptoms may originate from a combination of causes. The complaint of urethral discharge or dampness may be made by anxious patients who have become over-aware of genital sensation. Some patients complain of intermittent discharge: patients with mild urethritis may notice the discharge only in the morning or after urine has been retained for some hours, and patients with prostatorrhoea may notice the discharge only after defaecation. Patients with crystalluria may complain of 'chalky' discharge which occurs at the end of urination. Occasionally, discharge may be evident only by stains appearing on the underwear (although this symptom usually results from over-anxiety) or by a crust forming at the urinary meatus.

The history and examination will usually differentiate the anatomical origin of the discharge; occasionally differentiation is impossible because the patient has an unretractable prepuce (phimosis). Profuse, thick, purulent urethral discharge is likely to be caused by gonorrhoea; scanty, thin discharge is likely to be caused by non-gonococcal urethritis; subpreputial discharge is likely to be caused by balanoposthitis, often resulting from an elementary lack of hygiene but, if lumpy and irritant, it might be caused by candidiasis. The character of the discharge is a diagnostic clue but bacteriological examination is essential.

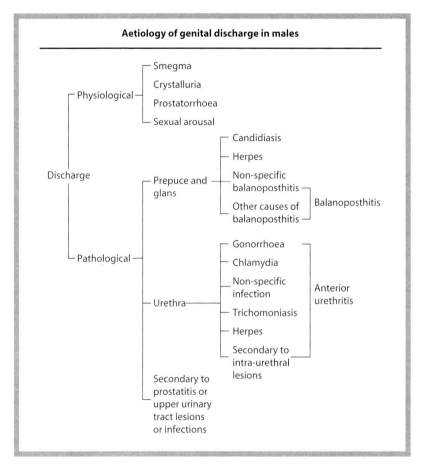

Aetiology of genital discharge in males

Discharge
- Physiological
  - Smegma
  - Crystalluria
  - Prostatorrhoea
  - Sexual arousal
- Pathological
  - Prepuce and glans
    - Candidiasis
    - Herpes
    - Non-specific balanoposthitis
    - Other causes of balanoposthitis
    } Balanoposthitis
  - Urethra
    - Gonorrhoea
    - Chlamydia
    - Non-specific infection
    - Trichomoniasis
    - Herpes
    } Anterior urethritis
    - Secondary to intra-urethral lesions
  - Secondary to prostatitis or upper urinary tract lesions or infections

↑ 35 Aetiology of genital discharge in males.

Urinary symptoms

Urinary symptoms are extremely variable and may originate from inflammatory conditions of the prepuce, meatus, anterior urethra or more proximal parts of the urinary tract, from crystalluria, or, in anxious patients, may occur without objective abnormal signs. The commonest symptoms are **pain** or **irritation** with urination; these are usually associated with meatitis or urethritis but can occur when urine comes in contact with an inflamed or fissured prepuce. Severe pain and scalding (traditionally 'like razor blades') is most often associated with gonococcal urethritis (see p. 120); acute retention occasionally develops in a primary episode of genital herpes and (rarely) in other forms of acute urethritis. Milder urethritis is more often associated with a complaint of irritation, initially located at the meatus but later passing proximally to the fossa navicularis and urethra. Usually pain and irritation are exacerbated by urination but are sometimes present at other times: symptoms are often most marked after urine has been retained for some hours or overnight. Suprapubic pain indicates cystitis or upper urinary tract involvement; perineal pain on urination or after ejaculation sometimes occurs in patients with prostatitis.

    Urgency and/or **frequency** of urination are common complaints which may occur alone (particularly in anxious individuals) or in association with other symptoms. These symptoms may be caused by meatitis or urethritis or may result from involvement of the proximal urinary tract or prostate.

    The early stages of urethritis or meatitis sometimes cause the edges of the urinary meatus to adhere so that the patient may notice difficulty in initiating urination, or that the urinary stream is split into several divergent pathways causing **spraying**; in patients who have experience of infection in the past this may be the first indication of trouble and the reason for attendance.

    Haematuria occasionally occurs: it is most frequently associated with cystitis, particularly with the condition known as acute haemorrhagic cystitis (see p. 139). Schistosomiasis should be considered in those recently in countries where the disease is endemic.

    Obstructive symptoms (difficulty in starting urination, poor stream, post-urination dribbling) are infrequent but, if present, may indicate involvement of the prostate or development of urethral stricture. Anxious patients are prone to complain of urinary dribbling or stained underwear following treatment but in most of these individuals no objective signs of persistent disease can be found.

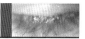

Aetiology of urinary symptoms in males

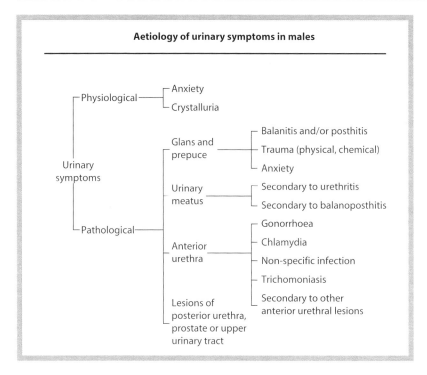

↑ **36 Aetiology of urinary symptoms in males.**

Scrotal symptoms

Symptoms originating from the scrotal area are relatively infrequent, and in many cases are not of pathological significance. Symptoms may originate from the surface or from within the scrotum; the cause may be local lesions or secondary to lesions elsewhere. Anxiety and attendance may be occasioned by the patient (often adolescent) becoming aware of a scrotal 'rash,' which on examination is found to be the normal or slightly prominent hair follicles and sebaceous glands, or by the discovery of a varicocele. Anxiety may be aroused by physiological activity of the dartos muscle: the resultant scrotal and testicular movement is thought to be abnormal.

The commonest scrotal symptom is complaint of a **rash** which is often pruritic. The rash may be localized or involve the whole scrotum and may also involve adjacent areas of the thigh, groin or penis. Scrotal cysts (see **20**) may enlarge and occasionally become infected. Other scrotal skin lesions are uncommon.

Symptoms arising inside the scrotum may result from conditions affecting the spermatic cord, the testicle and its coverings or the epididymis. The most common lesion of the spermatic cord likely to cause complaint is a cyst or spermatocele, but the cord may be tender or thickened in patients with epididymitis. **Painless swellings** within the scrotum are usually found to be hydroceles but the symptom may rarely be associated with other conditions such as tuberculosis, neoplastic disease or late syphilis. In tropical areas enormous scrotal swellings may occur in lymphogranuloma venereum (see p. 110) or filariasis but presentation at genitourinary clinics is unlikely. **Painful lesions** may originate from the epididymis or testis; differentiation is impossible on history and may be difficult on examination. The commonest painful lesion is epididymitis, usually secondary to urethritis or other urinary tract infections; inflammatory hydrocele is a common associated finding. Other causes of painful lesions are torsion of the testis (which is often a recurring condition) and mumps orchitis. Rarely, the development of epididymitis is the first symptom of gonococcal or other forms of urethritis.

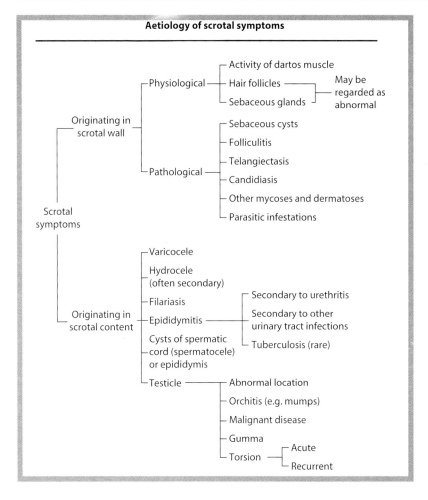

Aetiology of scrotal symptoms

↑ 37 Aetiology of scrotal symptoms.

Preputial symptoms

Preputial symptoms may be caused by local conditions affecting the glans penis and prepuce (balanoposthitis, see p. 192) or may be secondary to conditions originating elsewhere. Many patients with preputial symptoms have **phimosis** (see **16**), a condition which makes adequate hygiene and thorough examination difficult to achieve. The commonest complaints appearing to originate from the prepuce are those of discharge or urinary disorder; these have already been discussed (see pp. 26 and 28). Other common preputial symptoms are those designated **rash**, **cut** and **swelling**.

The term **rash** is frequently used to indicate erythema of the prepuce (and usually of the underlying glans) which may result from any of the causes of balanoposthitis or may refer to conditions such as genital warts or herpes. Pruritic erythema is often caused by candidiasis, fungal infection or hypersensitivity. Localized pruritic papules may be caused by scabies (see p. 230) or pruritic dermatoses such as lichen planus.

The term **cut** usually refers to small fissures appearing at the preputial margin, often following intercourse, or it may be used to describe ulcerative conditions. The symptom tends to be recurrent as the vicious circle arises of tissue damage/scarring/increased liability to further damage. Fissuring is common when phimosis is present and is often exacerbated by concomitant infections. It is frequently seen in patients with lichen sclerosus (LS) (see p. 222) and candidiasis (see p. 148).

Swelling (oedema) of the prepuce is frequently associated with trauma (often sexual activity) but may also occur with balanoposthitis or urethritis and is particularly marked if a phimotic prepuce is retracted and becomes caught behind the glans penis (paraphimosis, see **16**); oedema is usually more marked on the ventral surface.

Pale areas occurring at the preputial margin (often associated with phimosis) or patchily on other parts of the prepuce, penile shaft or glans penis may occasionally cause attendance. In most cases these lesions are caused by LS but (particularly in non-white patients) dyschromia may follow trauma or inflammatory conditions, or may arise from a congenital cause such as vitiligo.

Skin symptoms

Cutaneous symptoms originating from the prepuce, perineum and scrotum have already been discussed in preceding paragraphs, but symptoms may also originate from the pubis or penile shaft. In both these locations the commonest complaint is **rash**, which may be pruritic or non-pruritic. Contact dermatitis is discussed on page 241.

On the pubis, pruritic **rashes** are most often caused by parasitic infestations (pubic lice, see p. 228 or scabies, see p. 230) and often involve adjacent areas.

In scabies the itching is typically worse at night or when the patient is warm; in louse infestation the patient may notice nits attached to the hairs or the movement of parasites. Folliculitis, furunculosis and fungal infections may also cause pruritus. Rarely, other dermatoses such as lichen simplex (see p. 204) or lichen planus (see p. 206) may present as intensely pruritic pubic lesions. Injudicious self-application or ointments containing mercury compounds may sometimes cause a severe pruritic contact dermatitis (see **479**); history of such application should be sought in clinically suggestive cases. Anxiety is another cause of pubic pruritus; examination usually shows no abnormality, but sometimes patchy damage to pubic hairs caused by plucking or excoriation may be evident.

Non-pruritic pubic rash is a considerably less common complaint. Conditions such as molluscum contagiosum (see p. 183) may be found, or the term may be used in reference to warts or sebaceous cysts.

Pruritic and non-pruritic rash of the penile shaft is usually caused by one of the conditions discussed above. Occasionally a patient will attend complaining of vesicular lesions of the penile shaft; these are usually early lesions of herpes genitalis (see p. 167). The frequent complaint made by adolescents of **'rash'** on the penis is usually found to refer to the hair follicles and sebaceous glands on the ventral surface of the shaft which have only recently been noticed by the patient (see **11**).

Pigmentary changes affecting the pubis or penis are an occasional reason for attendance. Adolescents may become worried when the physiological increase in genital pigmentation at puberty is observed. Depigmentation may follow trauma or infection (particularly in non-white patients) or may be caused by lesions of LS/balanitis xerotica obliterans (see p. 222). In some patients pale macular lesions may be caused by tinea versicolor (see p. 202); lesions are usually more marked on the upper part of the body but rarely may be found solely on the genitalia. Haemangiomata may occur on the genitalia and be a source of anxiety (see **25**).

Perineal symptoms

Vague symptoms of **subcutaneous aching** and **mild discomfort** originating in the perineal region are fairly common. In the great majority of these cases no organic cause can be found; the symptoms of organic origin are most frequently caused by prostatitis (see p. 139) and may be associated with mild obstructive urinary symptoms. Genital herpetic infections are also prone to cause mild perineal discomfort. Rarely, acute prostatitis or acute cowperitis may cause severe deep perineal pain; perineal symptoms occasionally occur in cystitis or may be caused by referred pain from proctitis or anal lesions.

Lumps on the perineum are another occasional complaint. On examination, these may be found to be warts or sebaceous cysts (which may be infected) or in very rare cases abscesses originating in the urethra, prostate or Cowper's gland and pointing on the perineum.

Perineal pruritus can be caused by parasitic infestation, fungal infection or any intertriginous dermatosis. The possibility of contact dermatitis should not be forgotten.

Abnormalities of erection
Inadequate, absent or rapid loss of erection are the commonest complaints in this category. Anxiety or other psychological causes are by far the most likely cause of these symptoms; patients may attend an STD clinic with a belief that the phenomenon is related to previous transmissible infection.

Pain on erection or with ejaculation may occur in acute urethritis or may result from trauma sustained during sexual activity. Either of these symptoms may sometimes be the initial complaint in urethritis but in most cases the history and other findings make assessment of the complaint easy.

Curvature of the penis (**chordee**) during the erection is another symptom which may cause attendance. In most cases the complaint has no pathological significance but a small number of patients are found to have Peyronie's disease (see p. 245).

Priapism (persistent penile erection) is a symptom that occurs occasionally, but seldom alone. It is usually caused by urethritis or trauma (often resulting from sexual activity) but in rare cases may be caused by leukaemia or a crisis in sickle cell anaemia. It is also occasionally an unwanted side-effect of intracavernosal injection.

Bleeding
Complaint of frank bleeding is unusual but bloodstaining may be noticed with urethral discharge, ejaculation or as stains on clothing. Frank bleeding is nearly always associated with trauma, either accidental or occurring during sexual activity. The possibility of trauma associated with masturbation should not be forgotten. The commonest cause of bleeding is a tear of the fraenum causing haemorrhage (which is occasionally profuse) from the fraenal artery and vein. Traumatic haemorrhage from other genital sites may also occur; history is usually diagnostic. Bleeding is sometimes caused by upper urinary tract conditions, especially renal.

Scanty blood at the meatus may be the presenting symptom of

intraurethral warts; warts in other areas occasionally bleed after mild trauma. With severe urethritis and cystitis, bleeding may occur, almost always in association with urethral discharge or urinary symptoms.

Blood, often rusty or brown in colour, may be noticed in the ejaculate (**haematospermia**); this is a fairly frequent symptom in prostatitis (see p. 139) and may be the initial presentation. Haematospermia is a rare presentation of hypertension. The blood pressure should always be checked in patients with this symptom.

A few patients attend complaining of blood stains on the underwear. The cause may be one of those discussed above or it may be due to the minute bites of pubic lice; in the latter case examination of the underwear shows multiple pinpoints of dried blood.

FEMALE PATIENTS

Female patients may attend with symptoms or, more frequently, are totally asymptomatic and attend as a contact of a sexual partner already found to have transmissible disease. The evaluation of genital symptoms and the examination of asymptomatic attenders must always be comprehensive, and investigation with appropriate tests of all locations where evidence of disease may be found must be carried out. The findings are seldom so clearcut as to make diagnosis possible on clinical grounds alone, as the same symptoms and morphological appearance may be observed in conditions of differing aetiology. Even when symptoms are present, subjective factors in the individual patient influence the degree of complaint; findings on examination that appear identical to the doctor may be regarded as normal by one woman and abnormal by another. Further sources of confusion are lack of specificity in symptoms, the frequent finding that disease may affect several anatomical sites simultaneously, and the terminology used by patients. Paradoxically, it is also quite common for symptoms to be noticed only by their absence — after treatment the patient is aware of a change when previously ignored symptoms disappear.

In this subsection the significance of some of the more frequent symptoms is discussed in more detail. Inevitably there is considerable overlap. Concise tabulation of the aetiology of symptoms in female patients is difficult because of the mixture of symptomatology, anatomy and pathology. Our attempts at the analysis of symptoms are open to criticism from several aspects but are presented as indications of the aetiology of the more frequent complaints in adult patients. The conditions mentioned are more fully described later. No attempt has been made to include genitourinary disorders that mainly occur in paediatric or gynaecological practice. Ulcerative conditions have been discussed on page 20, lumps in the groin on page 22 and anogenital symptoms on page 24.

Bleeding

The most usual causes of the complaint of bleeding are trauma or lesions of the cervix. Less commonly, bleeding may result from gynaecological disorders (which are outside the scope of this book) or lesions of the vulva, urinary tract or vagina. The history is usually diagnostic when the bleeding is caused by trauma. Vulval ulceration, urethral caruncle, acute vaginitis and acute urinary tract infections may be the cause of the bleeding and with these conditions other symptoms are usually present. Ectopy of the cervix is frequently observed and may cause intermenstrual or postcoital bleeding; other cervical lesions such as ulceration, endometriosis or polyp may cause similar symptoms but are less common. Contraceptive methods must always be considered in any patient with this complaint—contraceptive agents (oral, injectable and depot) and intrauterine contraceptive devices are both fairly frequently associated with menstrual irregularity and intermenstrual spotting. It should not be forgotten that patients may use instruments or corrosive agents on themselves (often to procure abortion) and in these circumstances a truthful history may not be forthcoming.

Dyspareunia

Pain experienced during sexual intercourse (and occasionally with tampon usage) may result from physical or psychosexual factors, often in combination. The location of the pain is often diagnostically helpful: it may be at the introitus (superficial dyspareunia) or vaginal walls and/or in the pelvis (deep dyspareunia) or mixed. The most common physical cause is vulvitis, which is most likely to be caused by candidiasis, trichomioniasis or herpes. Other vulval lesions, such as inclusion cysts and hymenal tags, vestibulitis, contact dermatitis, previous surgery or infibulation, may also cause dyspareunia. Deficiency of the physiological mucous secretions may make intercourse painful. The deficiency may be caused by emotional factors, excessive washing or over-hasty intromission; atrophic changes may occur at and after the menopause; often when intercourse is attempted the resultant pain is likely to exacerbate the aridity.

Tenderness of the vaginal walls during intercourse may occur in patients with vaginitis. Pelvic pain on intercourse is a complaint of patients with salpingitis and endometritis (pelvic inflammatory disease—PID) or it may occur with gynaecological disorders such as ovarian cysts. The cervical excitation ('chandelier' sign) is positive when pelvic pain is provoked by movement of the cervix during bimanual examination. This is a feature of deep dyspareunia which is useful in the examination and evaluation of patients with complaint of pelvic pain.

Intrauterine contraceptive devices occasionally cause mild deep dyspareunia, and often cause colicky discomfort during menstruation; occasionally the irritable bowel syndrome or other intestinal problems may cause the symptoms.

Dyspareunia caused by psychosexual problems is often much more difficult to evaluate. When this diagnosis is suspected a detailed history may reveal a traumatic episode (e.g. sexual assault) preceding onset of the symptoms. If evaluation suggests that this type of problem is the likely cause of the complaint it is best, after physical causes have been excluded, to refer the patient (often together with the partner) to an experienced psychosexual counsellor.

Discharge

Discharge is a frequent complaint usually referring to an alteration of genital secretions which is regarded as excessive (a very subjective term) or abnormal by the patient. Discharge may be vulval, vaginal or cervical in origin and the cause may be physiological or pathological. In the history and examination, points to be particularly noted are the amount, colour and consistency of the discharge, the presence of abnormal odour, the presence of associated symptoms and relationship to the menstrual cycle or other specific factors such as sexual intercourse. Personal habits such as vaginal douching and antiseptic usage may cause discharge and relevant enquiry should be made. Evaluation of these points can be helpful in assessment but examination is always necessary to determine aetiology. There are numerous causes of discharge, but in practice most patients are found to have bacterial vaginosis (BV), candidiasis, trichomoniasis, gonorrhoea or non-gonococcal genital infection. **Pruritic discharge** is particularly associated with candidiasis; discharge with **'musty', 'foul' or 'fishy' odour** is most often caused by trichomoniasis, bacterial vaginosis or a vaginal foreign body; **bloodstained discharge** may be associated with disorders such as cervical erosion or metropathia, and may sometimes occur in acute trichomoniasis or herpes.

Vulval symptoms

Symptoms related by patients to the vulval region may, on analysis, be found to originate from the pubis, groin, perineum, upper thigh or vulva; a careful history is essential. Frequent symptoms are **pruritus**, **swelling**, **pain** or **'rash'**. Pruritus of the labia majora or pubis is usually caused by parasitic infestation; pruritus is almost invariable in symptomatic candidiasis but may result from any of the other causes of vulvitis. **Vulval swelling**, which is often exacerbated by coitus, is commonly caused by candidiasis but may be associated with trichomoniasis, herpes, syphilitic chancres or trauma. **Vulval pain** (and **superficial dyspareunia**, q.v.) may be intermittent or constant and is often related to urination or sexual intercourse. Vulvitis (particularly herpetic vulvitis) is the usual cause but lesions such as bartholinitis may be responsible. The term **'rash'** may refer either to inflammatory conditions of the skin or mucous membrane or, commonly, is a complaint made by patients who are found to have genital warts. Vulval symptoms may also extend to the perivulval areas such as the groin, perineum and natal cleft in candidiasis and onto the upper thigh in trichomoniasis. Vulval symptoms may also be caused by trauma or contact dermatitis, often due to careless or excessive use of soap (especially if perfumed) or antiseptics; specific enquiry should be made as the relevant history is often not volunteered. All these symptoms are highly variable in degree and should not be regarded as more than diagnostic clues, as none are pathognomonic.

'Lumps' of the vulva and adjacent areas are a frequent cause of complaint. The lumps may be physiological structures discovered during self-examination— hair follicles, sebaceous glands, varicosities and hymenal tags are examples of causes of this complaint, which are not pathological

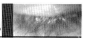
Aetiology of increased genital discharge in women

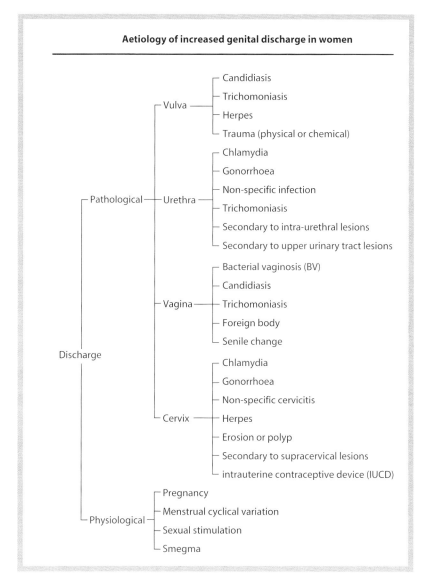

Discharge
- Pathological
  - Vulva
    - Candidiasis
    - Trichomoniasis
    - Herpes
    - Trauma (physical or chemical)
  - Urethra
    - Chlamydia
    - Gonorrhoea
    - Non-specific infection
    - Trichomoniasis
    - Secondary to intra-urethral lesions
    - Secondary to upper urinary tract lesions
  - Vagina
    - Bacterial vaginosis (BV)
    - Candidiasis
    - Trichomoniasis
    - Foreign body
    - Senile change
  - Cervix
    - Chlamydia
    - Gonorrhoea
    - Non-specific cervicitis
    - Herpes
    - Erosion or polyp
    - Secondary to supracervical lesions
    - intrauterine contraceptive device (IUCD)
- Physiological
  - Pregnancy
  - Menstrual cyclical variation
  - Sexual stimulation
  - Smegma

↑ **38 Aetiology of increased genital discharge in women.**

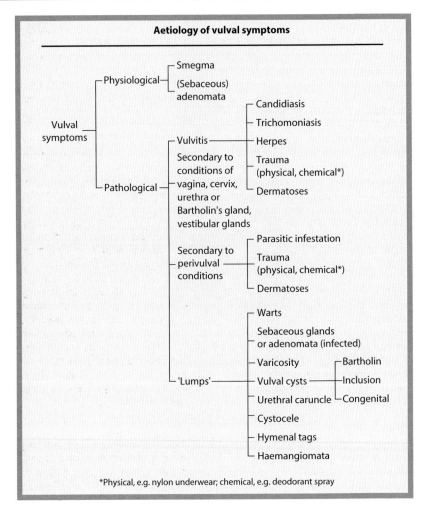

Aetiology of vulval symptoms

↑ **39 Aetiology of vulval symptoms.**

conditions but may be a source of anxiety. Painless lumps, such as vulval or perivulval haemangiomata, epidermal inclusion cysts, Gartner's duct cysts and Bartholin's cysts, may also cause the patient to seek advice. Cystocele, cysts of Skene's glands and urethral lesions, such as caruncle or prolapsed mucosa, may be found to be the reason for the complaint. Genital warts (see p. 185) are frequently first noticed as lumpy growths on the labia or vulva. Bruises resulting from trauma (sometimes during intercourse) may be noticed as painful lumps, and other painful lesions include pyogenic skin conditions such as furunculosis or abscess.

Urinary symptoms

Urinary symptoms are very variable and are never pathognomonic. Complaint may be made of **urgency**, **discomfort** or **pain** associated with urination, **upper urinary tract symptoms** and, rarely, retention. In addition patients often complain of an alteration in **urinary odour** (the term 'strong' is often used) or may notice a change in colour which may result from alteration in specific gravity, blood (haematuria), or metabolites of drugs which are excreted in the urine. Symptoms may be caused by lesions of the vulva, urethra, bladder or upper urinary tract; a detailed history is most helpful in analysis. **Pain** or **discomfort** on urination confined to the meatus or vulva is usually associated with vulval conditions, urethral caruncle or urethritis, whereas the same symptoms associated with frequency, urgency or strangury are more likely to be caused by cystitis or upper urinary tract infection or, occasionally, by referred symptoms in patients with cervicitis. **Severe dysuria** and **acute retention** may be caused by urethra or vulval ulceration and are most commonly seen in first attacks of herpes. Appraisal of the complain of **haematuria** must also consider other origins for blood seen at the vulva or in the voided urine, such as menstruation or bleeding lesions of the vagina or supravaginal structures in the upper urinary tract.

Skin symptoms

Most symptoms originating from vulval cutaneous tissues have already been discussed in the paragraphs referring to discharge and vulval symptomatology but some patients present with symptoms originating on the pubis. The aetiology of this symptom is similar in male and female patients and the reader is referred to page 32. In practice, it is noticeable that females appear much less likely to become anxious about skin symptoms when these are the sole abnormality present; most female patients who mention skin symptoms have other symptoms which are the main reason for attendance. An occasional reason for the complaint of **'rash'** of the vulva are the minute, branny, sebaceous glands of the glabrous interlabial surfaces which may be found (and considered abnormal) by patients during self-examination.

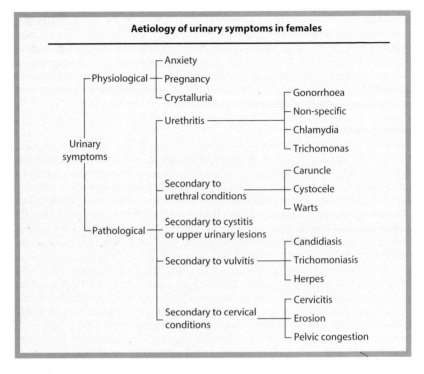

↑ 40 Aetiology of urinary symptoms in females.

Odour

Complaint of abnormal genital odour is frequently made and may be the only complaint, but more commonly it is associated with other symptoms such as vaginal discharge. The abnormal odour may be described as **'sour'** or **'acid'** when candidiasis is present; a **'foul'**, **'musty'** or **'fishy'** odour is typically associated with trichomoniasis or bacterial vaginosis. Retained vaginal foreign bodies (often tampons) and necrotic lesions of the vagina or cervix may cause an extremely unpleasant 'faecal' odour.

Abdominal pain

Abdominal pain resulting from lower genitourinary tract disease is a relatively infrequent complaint in practice, but is occasionally the sole reason for presentation. **It must always be remembered that patients who are anxious about 'VD' may attend a clinic with abdominal pain which has a non-venereal cause: conditions such as irritable bowel syndrome or gynaecological disorders should be appropriately referred**. **Mild aching** and **discomfort** in the lower abdomen and groins may occur with any genitourinary pathology but is common in patients with acute vaginitis or herpetic infection. Cystitis (which may result from infection ascending from the urethra) is another common cause of lower abdominal pain encountered in practice; pain is usually suprapubic and intermittent and is often exacerbated by urination. Salpingitis (PID) may be the presenting feature in patients with gonorrhoea or non-gonococcal genital infection; sometimes pain is felt only on intercourse (**deep dyspareunia** q.v.) but more commonly the pain, of variable severity, is felt in one or both iliac fossae and is colicky and intermittent, but may be persistent. In patients with endometriosis, pain is usually central and may be referred to the rectum or anus or to the groin: deep dyspareunia and abnormalities of menstruation are usual. Assessment of the complaint of pain requires careful analysis of the findings from the history and examination including ultrasound.

TECHNIQUES OF EXAMINATION

INTRODUCTION

Many people attending an STD clinic for the first time are, understandably, extremely apprehensive and it is essential that the rooms in which patients are interviewed and examined are quiet, private and well-illuminated.

HIV-associated problems (or anxiety concerning these problems) are now increasingly common in practice. At present, serological examination for HIV antibodies is not undertaken routinely in the UK: in appropriate circumstances, after counselling, blood samples can be sent for examination. Reattendance is arranged to discuss the results and any follow-up or further consultation.

Full clinical examination will often be necessary as genital symptoms and lesions are often caused by systemic disease. Complete genital examination is always necessary, and particular attention should be directed to remote sites where lesions that are helpful in the diagnosis of genital disorders may often be found. These remote sites include the eyes and conjunctivae, the oral cavity and pharynx, the skin and nails and the lymphatic system. Examination will usually include taking specimens for laboratory tests.

The diagnosis and management of many conditions encountered in genitourinary practice is often facilitated by the use of appropriate haematological and biochemical techniques. The changing pattern of morbidity is reflected in the types of examination requested: for example, many clinicians in industrialized countries now think that serological tests for syphilis should be undertaken, e.g. in ante-natal clinics, only when indicated rather than as a routine. The authors remain in favour of routine screening.

Genital examination of male patients

The external genitalia, pubis and inguinal regions are inspected for superficial lesions or glandular enlargement.

The shaft of the penis is palpated, and the condition of the testes, epididymides and spermatic cords is also assessed by palpation.

The prepuce (if present) is examined and retractability assessed. In some patients contraction of the preputial margin (phimosis) may make reflection of the prepuce impossible; in rare cases, surgical incision of the prepuce (dorsal slit) may be necessary to allow adequate examination (see **41**).

Examination of the glans penis, the coronal sulcus and subpreputial sac is made with the prepuce reflected: if balanitis or balanoposthitis is present, bacteriological specimens are taken.

The external urinary meatus is examined. If urethral discharge is present it may be visible or expressed by digital massage along the line of the urethra. It is preferable that urine should be retained for several hours before urethral examination—if urination has been recent urethral discharge may not have had sufficient time to accumulate. Suitable bacteriological specimens are taken.

The perineum, anus and perianal regions are inspected. In anoreceptive homosexuals proctoscopy and bacteriological examination are necessary. Digital examination of the prostate gland may be required, but the procedure is usually performed later. Inspection of the distal urethra can be made with a modified otoscope (meatoscope).

If genital ulcer disease is found, suitable examination specimens are taken. At the conclusion of examination the patient should be requested to pass urine for the 'two glass' test (see p. 52) and for testing to exclude abnormal urinary constituents.

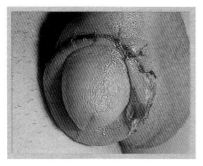

↑ 41 Dorsal slit.

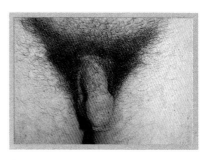

↑ 42 The abdomen, genitalia, groins and thighs are inspected.

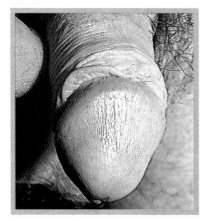

← 43 The prepuce is retracted.

Urethral and subpreputial examination of male patients

Apparatus. Microscope slides and cover slips. Disposable plastic loop or other suitable swab, and culture swabs. Culture and/or transport media. Saline. Cleansing swabs. Gloves for examiner.

Technique. The prepuce (if present) is reflected. In cases of balanitis or balanoposthitis the specimens are taken from the preputial sac. In suspected urethritis the glans penis is cleaned and the specimens taken from the urethral orifice with the plastic loop or swab. For stained smears, the specimen is spread thinly on a glass slide and allowed to dry. For smears to examine for *Trichomonas vaginalis* the specimen taken is mixed with a drop of saline on the slide and the drop is then covered with a cover slip (NB: this technique has low sensitivity).

Cultures are taken with suitable swabs. The specimens may either be inoculated directly on to or into a suitable medium or the specimens may be placed in transport medium for transmission to the laboratory.

Ulcerated lesions usually require examination by dark-ground microscopy; the technique is described on page 49. Occasionally other diagnostic methods are used.

Proctoscopy is undertaken for anoreceptive homosexuals (see p. 50).

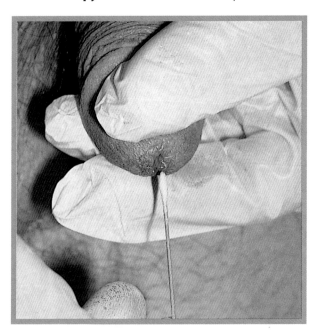

← 44 Taking an urethral swab.

Genital examination of female patients

Examination is most easily conducted with the patient in the lithotomy position. Good lighting, with an adjustable lamp, is essential.

The external genitalia, pubis and anal region are inspected and the groins palpated. Any enlargement of Bartholin's glands is noted and the presence of urethral or vaginal discharge is also noted. The labia should be carefully separated and the clitoral hood reflected for adequate examination. Ulcerative lesions should be appropriately investigated.

A speculum of suitable size and design (e.g. Cusco) is gently introduced through the introitus and passed into the vagina to expose the cervix. If lubrication of the instrument is necessary to facilitate introduction, this should be done with water or saline, as the use of other lubricants may interfere with subsequent bacteriology. The vaginal walls and cervix are inspected and bacteriological specimens taken. Occasionally, removal of foreign bodies is necessary.

After dry-swabbing of the cervix and inspection, endocervical bacteriological specimens are taken, and smears for cervical exfoliative cytology may also be taken. The latter may be performed at initial examination, but in many clinics this is not done until any infection present (which may make interpretation of the smear difficult) has been treated. Testing with 5% acetic acid and/or Lugol's iodine can be undertaken.

After withdrawal of the speculum, the urethral meatus is inspected and bacteriological specimens taken. If findings indicate the need, bacteriological specimens are taken from lesions of Bartholin's glands or Skene's glands.

Proctoscopy and examination of rectal smears and cultures may be helpful, but this procedure is not usually done routinely. This investigation may be particularly helpful in patients suspected of gonorrhoea or threadworm infestation (see p. 50).

Bimanual pelvic examination is undertaken to assess the uterus and other pelvic organs. Inspection and palpation of the abdomen concludes the examination.

The patient is requested to pass urine, which is then tested for the presence of abnormal constituents or may be sent for laboratory examination.

Urethral, vaginal, cervical and rectal examination of female patients

Apparatus. As for urethral examination in male patients (see p. 46). Vaginal speculae. Sponge-holding forceps. Proctoscope and lubricant. Gloves for examiner.

Technique. The vaginal speculum is passed to expose the vaginal vault and the cervix; the vaginal walls are inspected. With a plastic loop or cotton-tipped swab, material is taken from the pool of vaginal secretion in the posterior fornix — this material is used to make preparations for staining and for examination for *Trichomonas vaginalis* and other vaginal pathogens. The external surface of the cervix is cleansed with a dry swab and specimens are taken from within the cervical canal. Cervical cytology can also be undertaken.

Specimens from the urethra are taken in a similar manner; usually a specimen for staining is the only requirement, but saline drop preparations for *T. vaginalis* may be necessary. If specimens are required from Bartholin's glands or Skene's glands, these are prepared in the same way.

Proctoscopy is performed to inspect the anal canal and rectum and for specimens to be taken.

Cultures are taken from the same sites and are either plated directly on to or into suitable media or placed in transport medium.

Ulcerated lesions usually need to be examined by dark-ground microscopy or other methods (see p. 49).

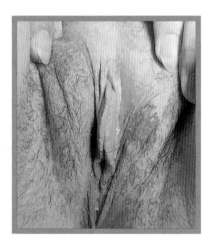

↑ 45 Inspection of the vulva
The patient has herpes.

↑ 46 Inspection of the cervix and vaginal vault.

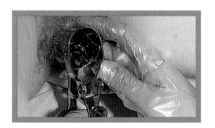

← 47 Introduction of Cusco speculum.

Ulcerated lesions

The aetiology of ulcerated genital lesions is protean, but early syphilis is the most important disease to exclude. In this disease, the microscopical examination of specimens with **dark-ground** (or **dark-field**) illumination is essential. Other diagnostic methods (e.g. other bacteriology, biopsy, etc.) may be used but these are not detailed here. Dark-field examination may have to be repeated on several occasions or on several consecutive days before a firm diagnosis can be made: no treponemicidal therapy should be used until examinations are completed.

Apparatus. Glass slides and cover slips (thin slides are most suitable). Scarifiers: a cotton swab is often suitable but a metal instrument may be used. Capillary tubes. Gloves for examiner.

Technique. The lesion is cleaned with normal saline to remove surface debris. The surface is scarified and then the base of the ulcer gently squeezed so that serum exudes onto the surface. This serum is collected on the edge of a cover slip, which is then placed in the centre of a slide. The preparation is compressed to produce a thin film which is immediately examined microscopically. If microscopic facilities are not immediately available, serum may be collected in a capillary tube. The ends of the capillary tube are sealed and the tube sent to the laboratory for examination; in such preparations *T. pallidum* can survive for several days (see **48**).

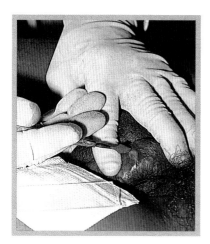

← 48 Dark-field microscopy
Scarifying lesions with metal scarifier.

Gland aspiration (gland puncture)

This technique may be used to obtain material for dark-ground microscopical examination and other bacteriological examination in cases when such material is unobtainable from the ulcerated lesion but enlarged regional lymph nodes are present (see **49**). A similar technique is sometimes used to collect material from the edge of healing ulcers.

Apparatus. Syringe and intramuscular needle. Thin glass slides and cover slips. Sterile saline. Skin disinfectant. Gloves for examiner.

Technique. The skin is disinfected. A minute quantity of saline is aspirated into the needle. The needle is introduced into the gland and the saline expelled. The gland is gently massaged over the tip of the needle and the syringe is aspirated. After withdrawal from the gland the material in the needle is expelled onto a slide and covered with a cover slip. The preparation is compressed and examined microscopically.

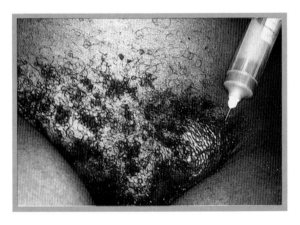

← 49 Gland aspiration
The patient has LGV (lymphogranuloma venereum). A similar technique is used in diagnostic aspiration.

Proctoscopy

Proctoscopy is essential in the examination of anoreceptive homosexual patients and is often used in the diagnosis of gonorrhoea in female patients. In addition, proctoscopy may be helpful in the evaluation of patients suspected of having syphilis, lymphogranuloma venereum or genital warts, and occasionally in other conditions.

Apparatus. Disposable proctoscope (an instrument with built-in illumination is preferable). Lubricant. Plastic loop or cotton-tipped swab. Culture and/or transport media. Glass slides and cover slips. Gloves for examiner.

Technique. Female patients are examined in lithotomy or lateral positions. Male patients may be examined in either a kneeling position or the lateral position. The lubricated proctoscope (with obturator *in situ*) is gently pressed against the anus and inserted into the rectum; it is often helpful if the patient is asked to push backwards against the instrument during introduction. The obturator is removed and the rectum inspected: bacteriological or other specimens may be taken. The instrument is slowly withdrawn while the distal part of the rectum and anal canal is observed (see **50**).

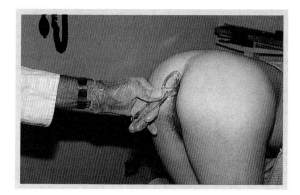

← **50 Proctoscopy.**

Urine tests

All patients should have urine specimens tested for the presence of abnormal constituents such as protein, glucose and blood. Microscopical examination of urine may be necessary to determine the nature of crystal deposits which may occasionally cause symptoms of urethritis. In rare cases, ova of *Schistosoma haematobium* may be found. In cases of suspected upper urinary tract infection, midstream or clean specimens of urine should be sent to the laboratory for microscopy and bacterial culture.

Male patients. The **'two glass'** test is a useful clinical indication in the assessment of the site of infection and in examination after treatment of urethritis.

The patient is given two urine glasses and requested to pass 50–60 ml into the first glass and the remainder into the second glass. Debris from any anterior urethral inflammation present will be voided with the first specimen and the second glass will contain urine representative of the contents of the bladder. The test is not completely reliable and the findings may be unrepresentative in very severe cases of anterior urethritis and in cases when the urine has been retained only for a short time before testing.

← **51 Two glass test.**

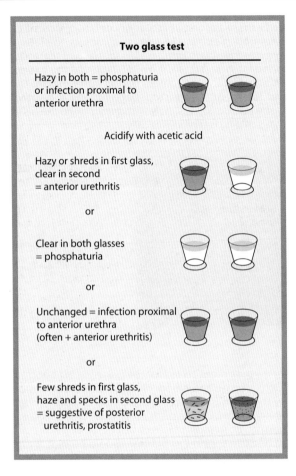

Two glass test

Hazy in both = phosphaturia
or infection proximal to
anterior urethra

Acidify with acetic acid

Hazy or shreds in first glass,
clear in second
= anterior urethritis

or

Clear in both glasses
= phosphaturia

or

Unchanged = infection proximal
to anterior urethra
(often + anterior urethritis)

or

Few shreds in first glass,
haze and specks in second glass
= suggestive of posterior
  urethritis, prostatitis

The prostate gland and prostatic massage

Examination of the prostate may reveal chronic prostatitis or the now rare acute prostatitis or prostatic abscess. Cowperitis and vesiculitis may also be detected by rectal examination, but these are also rare conditions.

Examination of the prostatic (or prostatovesicular) secretion expressed by digital massage of the gland was formerly a common procedure in tests of cure after treatment of urethritis. At present the technique is still occasionally used for this purpose but is more frequently used in the investigation of persistent urethritis or other genital symptoms and in conditions such as uveitis and Reiter's syndrome, or in the treatment of chronic prostatitis.

The significance of abnormal findings in prostatic fluid remains a matter of controversy.

Apparatus. Gloves and lubricant. Glass slides and cover slips. Culture and/or transport media (rarely required).

Technique of prostatic massage. The patient should be in either the knee–elbow position or bending over a low chair. A lubricated gloved finger is introduced into the rectum and the prostate and seminal vesicals palpated. Prostatic fluid is expressed by digital massage (see **52**) and collected at the urethral orifice for microscopic or bacteriological examination. It may be necessary to 'milk' the urethra to express the fluid. Massage should not be done in the presence of acute prostatic infection because of the risk of bacteraemia.

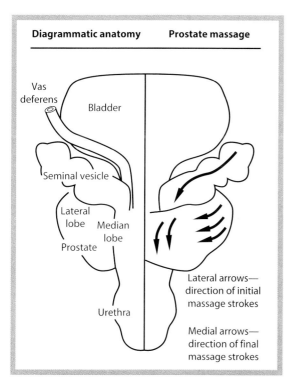

← 52 Prostatic massage.

Anterior urethroscopy

Direct visual examination of the anterior urethra is most often used when urethral stricture or urethral infiltration is suspected. The technique may also be used in the investigation of cases of persistent urethritis, or when **littritis** or another intraurethral lesion is thought to be present. Occasionally intraurethral surgical techniques may be performed with the urethroscope. In the past, anterior urethroscopy to exclude stricture was a part of the test of cure after treatment or urethritis, but this complication is now so rare that routine urethroscopy is seldom practised. The instrument may also be used for vaginal examination in infants.

Apparatus. Anterior urethroscope (the instrument consists of a cannula with obturator to which may be attached a lighting system, a telescope and air distension system). Urethral anaesthetic. Penile clamp. Disinfectant. Gloves for examiner.

Technique. Strict sterile precautions must be observed; with rare exceptions, the examination is not carried out while acute urethritis is present. After cleansing and sterilization of the glans penis, local anaesthetic is introduced and massaged down the urethra. The penile clamp is applied until the anaesthetic has taken effect. The lubricated cannula of the urethroscope (with obturator in place) is gently passed down the urethra as far as it will comfortably go. The obturator is withdrawn and the light and telescope fittings are attached. After the telescope has been focused, the urethra is distended by air pressure and the epithelium observed; normal epithelium has a glistening and pink appearance. The urethroscope is slowly withdrawn while the walls are kept under observation. Oedema or strictures may be found; when littritis is present, the intraurethral duct orifices are infected and swollen and show up as dark dots.

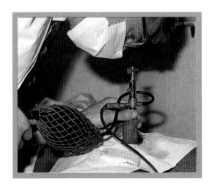

← **53 Urethroscopy.**

Colposcopy

The colposcope is increasingly being used in genitourinary medicine. It is a low-power binocular microscope (×10 to ×40) with a focal length of around 30 cm (12 in) which is used to examine lesions or structures in detail and (when appropriate) enables biopsy specimens to be taken with precision. The colposcope is of particular value in examining the cervix, which is so often involved in HPV infections (see p. 186). Many patients who would previously have been referred to the gynaecologist can now be dealt with within the department, but it is extremely important that staff in genitourinary clinics should work closely with their gynaecological colleagues.

The instrument may also occasionally be of great value in the examination of other genital lesions.

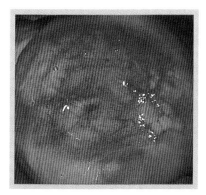

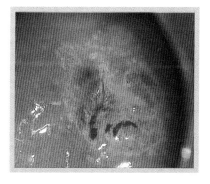

← 54 Cervical ectropion (pronounced)
This is a variation of normal appearance in women of reproductive age, who are either on the oral contraceptive pill or pregnant.

↑ 56 Appearance of cervical wart after application of acetic acid
Clearly demarcated area of acetowhite with some contact bleeding after application of acetic acid.

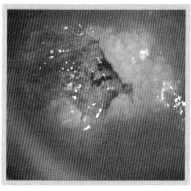

↑ 55 Cervical wart.

Collection of blood specimens

Examination of blood specimens is often extremely helpful in diagnosis and management. However, it is important to remember that some specimens are in themselves hazardous (e.g. in patients with hepatitis B or HIV) and laboratory investigation should be requested only when the result will clearly be of help in case management; **it is essential that such specimens are clearly labelled conforming to local laboratory policy.**

Apparatus. Sterile dry syringes, needles and collecting tubes (alternative: vacuum venesection). Tourniquet. Skin disinfectant. Stylets for heel stabs in infants. Gloves for phlebotomist; 'high risk' labels.

Technique. In adults it is usually easy to collect blood by venepuncture in the antecubital fossa. A tourniquet is placed round the limb proximal to the vein selected. The skin is disinfected. The vein is steadied and the needle inserted. Blood is aspirated into the syringe or vacuum tube and the tourniquet is released before the needle is withdrawn. Digital pressure will control any bleeding from the puncture. The blood in the syringe is expelled into the collecting tube after the needle has been removed: if the blood is expelled through the needle haemolysis may occur and invalidate subsequent examination.

In infants it is easiest to collect specimens by heel stab (see **57**). The stylet is used and the specimen collected in a capillary or other collecting tube. Other sites for venepuncture include scalp veins and the central sinus.

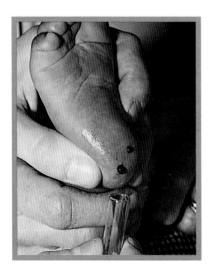

← 57 Heel stab in infant.

Other techniques
Many other methods of investigation may occasionally be used in STD clinics. These investigations may be indicated by the history given by the patient or by the clinical examination.

KOH: Amine ('sniff test'). A loopful of vaginal secretion is mixed with a drop of 10% KOH on a slide. When bacterial vaginosis is present a characteristic odour is produced, detected by sniffing.
   The technique can also be used to demonstrate by microscopy fungal elements in skin scrapings or vaginal discharge.

Lumbar puncture. Indicated in cases of neurosyphilis or to exclude asymptomatic neurosyphilis. It is also increasingly used in HIV to make specific diagnoses (see **579** and **581**).

Radiology. Indicated in syphilis when skeletal lesions or aortitis are suspected Indicated in conditions such as Reiter's syndrome or other arthritides. Often indicated in HIV (see page 283). **Ultrasound** and other imaging techniques may be of great help especially in the investigation of patients suspected of having pelvic inflammatory disease (**PID**), patients with testicular problems and patients with prostatitis.

Skin tests. Indicated in suspected contact dermatitis and some other dermatoses. Occasionally indicated in HIV disease complications, such as tuberculosis.

Slit-lamp microscopy. Indicated in suspected congenital syphilis to exclude previous interstitial keratitis, and in the management of uveitis which may occur in conditions such as Reiter's syndrome.

Laparoscopy (direct visual inspection of the pelvis) is often helpful in the evaluation of patients with abdominal pain. This examination is undertaken by gynaecologists: for further information the reader is referred to appropriate textbooks.

The investigative methods referred to above are the most frequently used; there are, of course, many others that may be used from time to time, especially **endoscopy**.

THE TREPONEMAL DISEASES

The treponemal diseases (the **treponematoses**) are a group of conditions which are caused by organisms at present morphologically and serologically indistinguishable, but which have different clinical patterns. It seems probable that the clinical patterns observed today result from the adaption to environmental changes, over the ages, of a common ancestral organism.

Venereal (sexual) and **non-venereal** transmission may occur. The non-venereal treponematoses are usually designated **benign**, since late complications and congenital transmission are either unimportant, rare or unknown.

Classification
The treponematoses may be classified by the usual mode of transmission:
- Venereal transmission: **syphilis**
- Non-venereal transmission: **endemic syphilis**, **yaws**, **pinta**

Many other non-venereal treponematoses have been nosologically differentiated, usually by local dialect names; these conditions probably represent varieties of endemic syphilis (see p. 100).

Distribution
Syphilis: worldwide.
Endemic syphilis: formerly widespread, now seen almost entirely in areas of low socioeconomic status.
Yaws: humid tropical areas.
Pinta: central America and non-western areas of South America.

The organism
Treponema pallidum was identified as the cause of syphilis by Schaudinn and Hoffman in 1905. Morphologically, the organism is a slender spiral with regular coils and tapering ends. The number of coils is usually between 10 and 15 and the organism's length is about 8 μm, though an organism may be shorter or longer with less or more coils. Its diameter is about 0.25 μm. Electron microscopy shows an axial bundle of fine fibrils surrounded by a narrow capsule. Division is usually by transverse fission, which occurs at intervals of 30–36 hours. It seems probable that cyst forms can occur (see **58** and **59**). *T. pertenue* and *T. carateum* cannot be distinguished from *T. pallidum*.

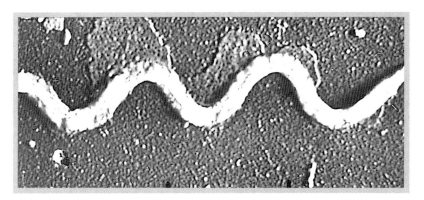

↑ 58 Electron photomicrograph of *Treponema pallidum.*

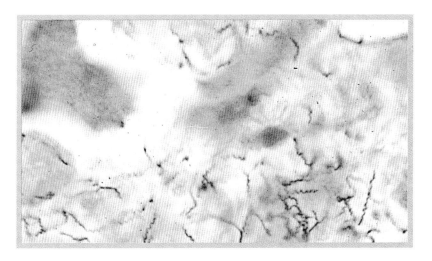

↑ 59 *Treponema pallidum* Stained fetal liver.

SYPHILIS

Syphilis is a contagious disease caused by *Treponema pallidum.* It is a systemic disease which, when untreated, has overt and covert phases. The diagram below (**60**) outlines the progress of the untreated infection.

Syphilis is usually acquired by sexual contact but untreated pregnant women may pass infection through the placenta to the fetus (congenital syphilis). It is occasionally acquired through non-sexual means (e.g. in medical or laboratory workers in contact with infectious patients or the organism, through transfusion of blood from an infected donor to a susceptible recipient and, very rarely, through inanimate objects). Spirochaetaemia and the distribution of the organism throughout the body occur before clinical lesions appear.

Diagnosis of syphilis

The diagnostic methods used depend on the stage of the disease at the time of presentation; these are discussed in the relevant subsections.

Recognition of *T. pallidum*. The only practical method (for clinical use) of demonstrating *T. pallidum* is by dark-ground microscopy. The organism is so slender that when stained by histological methods rapid enough for routine clinic usage it is not differentiated. Microscopy using transmitted light may be used when preparations are stained by silver impregnation. This method is suitable for biopsy specimens but is impractical for routine use. Culture on artificial media is unsuccessful. Experimentally, the organism will live and reproduce in suitable animal innoculations but culture is not a clinical practicality. Techniques using fluorescent staining methods have been developed for clinical use, but sensitivity is too low for routine clinical use.

Dark-ground microscopy. The technique of preparing a specimen for dark-ground (dark-field) microscopy is described on page 49.

Syphilis is recognized as a thin silver spiral which is motile, actively angulating and often undulating. The organism may rotate, and the length may vary as the coils compress and expand like a spring. Differentiation has to be made from other spiral organisms (e.g. *Treponema refringens*). The morphological appearances and the patterns of movements of other organisms are different and, with experience, the distinction is usually simple.

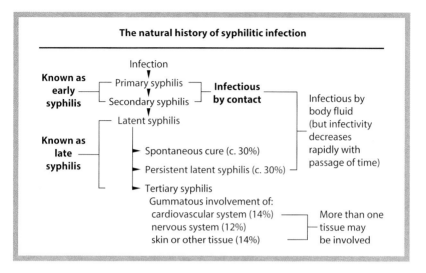

The natural history of syphilitic infection

↑ 60 The natural history of syphilitic infection.

Serological tests for syphilis (STS). There are many different tests for syphilis differing in sensitivity, in specificity and in convenience of use. The most usual tests in practice are the non-specific Venereal Disease Research Laboratory (VDRL) slide test, the specific test *Treponema pallidum* Haemagglutination (TPHA) and the Fluorescent *Treponema* Antibody (FTA) test; the *Treponema pallidum* Immobilisation (TPI) test is accurate but technically difficult and time-consuming and is therefore now seldom used. The FTA test using specific immunoglobulin fractions shows that IgM can be found before the clinical lesion appears: IgG is found shortly afterwards and persists for long periods, even after treatment. There is some evidence to suggest that when IgM is found the disease is active. If this is confirmed, the significance of a positive STS will be easier to evaluate. The various stages of syphilitic infection show different patterns of reaction, summarized below:

Patterns of syphilitic reaction

	Primary <30 days	Primary >30 days	Secondary	Latent	Late	Treated
VDRL	–	+	+ ➔ +++ (may be titrated)	+ or ±	+ ➔ ++	± or –
TPHA	–	–	+	+	+	+
FTA	±	+	++	+	+	+, ± or –

↑ **61 The various stages of syphilitic infection**
show different patterns of reaction, summarized above.

Screening is often undertaken with a simple test (e.g. VDRL); doubtful or positive results are rechecked in a different specimen and with the addition of a more specific/sensitive test (TPHA, FTA). The possibility of a prozone reaction with the VDRL test should be remembered: strongly positive sera may give misleading negative results when tested only at low titres.

Evaluation of positive serological tests for syphilis (STS). In practice, one of the common problems that occurs is the evaluation of the patient with normal findings on clinical examination but who has positive STS and originates from an area where treponematosis is endemic. It is impossible to determine with certainty whether positive results are residual from treponemal disease acquired in childhood or are from venereally acquired syphilis. In practice, in the absence of verifiable information, it is probably best to investigate and treat the patient as a case of latent syphilis.

Primary syphilis

The lesion is traditionally known as the **primary chancre**. Primary syphilis is the clinical stage of the disease when the infection first becomes manifest as a lesion of skin or mucous membrane. Most lesions (95 %) occur on, or adjacent to, the external genitalia. Lesions may be concealed (e.g. intraurethral, rectal, cervical and anal lesions); the patient is often unaware that infection is present. Other areas of sexual contact (e.g. mouth, nipple) may be the location of extragenital lesions and other extragenital lesions may be the result of non-sexual infection in medical and other workers in contact with the disease or organism.

Incubation period

The time between infection and the appearance of the primary lesion is usually between 21 and 35 days, but the lesion may occur any time between 10 and 90 days after infection.

Clinical presentation

The primary lesion (**chancre**) begins as a small dusky red macule which soon develops into a papule. The surface of the papule erodes to form an ulcer which is typically round and painless, with a clean surface. The base of the lesion is indurated and feels firm or hard on palpation. Often considerable oedema of adjacent tissues is present. Untreated, the ulcer pursues an indolent course, slowly enlarging to about 2 cm in diameter and then slowly healing, usually without residual scarring, after 4–8 weeks. In about 50% of cases, a single chancre is present; in the remainder, multiple but similar lesions, often 'kissing', are found; confluence may occur. Regional lymph gland enlargement (**syphilitic bubo**) begins 1–2 weeks after the appearance of the primary chancre. On palpation, affected glands are felt to be firm, discrete and slightly to moderately enlarged. Gland involvement may be painless but a proportion of affected patients complain of aching and/or tenderness of the involved glands. In clinical practice, about 50% of patients found to have primary syphilis have a syphilitic bubo.

Following treatment, the primary chancre heals very quickly: it stops being infectious within 24 hours of starting effective treponemicidal therapy. If a bubo is present when treatment is begun, resolution of the glands may take several months.

Diagnosis

Diagnosis is made by demonstration of *T. pallidum* (see p. 59) by dark-ground microscopy in material taken from the suspect lesion. Clinical diagnosis is inadequate as many primary chancres have an **atypical** appearance and other conditions can mimic primary syphilis.

Serological examination is essential. About 60% of patients with primary syphilis are found to have positive reactions: in patients who are found to have negative serological tests, the infection has been present for too short a time for antibody to reach detectable levels (see p. 62).

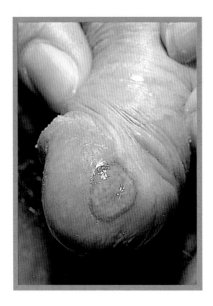

↑ **62 Primary chancre**
of glans penis.

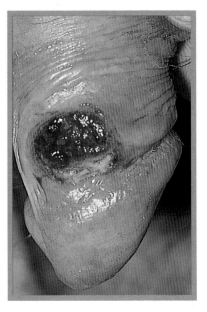

↑ **63 Primary chancre.**

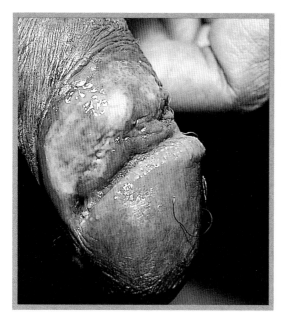

← 64 Extensive ulceration in primary syphilis
Note absence of secondary infection.

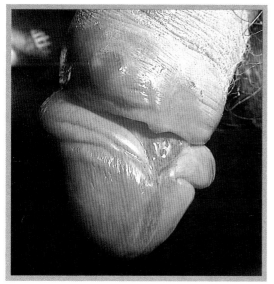

← 65 Primary chancre.

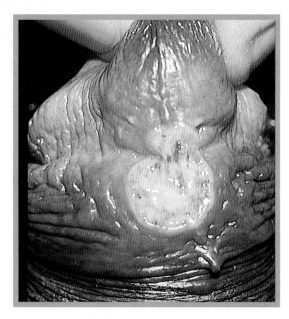

← **66 Extensive 'kissing' chancres** of frenum.

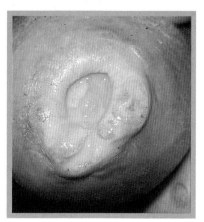

↑ **67 Multiple small chancres** associated with phimosis and secondary infection.

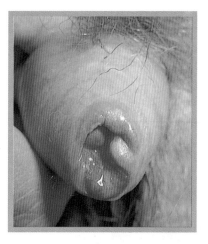

↑ **68 Chancre of fissured, phimotic prepuce.**

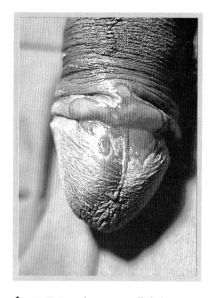

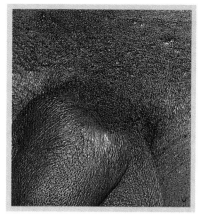

↑ 70 'Condom' chancre
Note pubic molluscum.

↑ 69 Extensive superficial chancres
The lesions were not indurated.

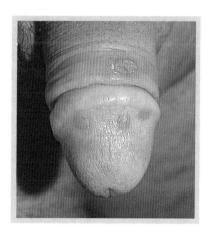

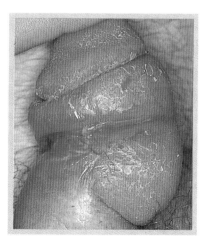

↑ 72 Chancre with extensive cellulitis and oedema
(see **466**, 'saxophone' penis).

↑ 71 Multiple primary chancres.

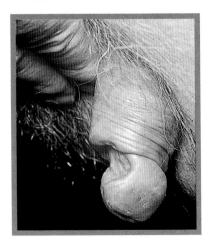

↑ **73 Penile scarring**
following primary syphilis.
Infrequently seen.

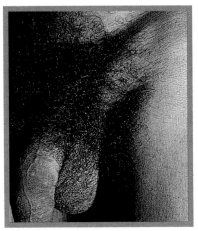

↑ **74 Syphilitic bubo.**

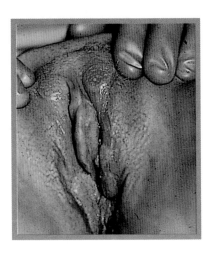

↑ **75 'Kissing' chancres of labia majora.**

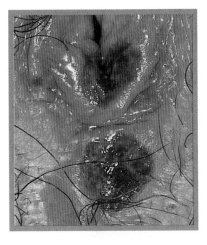

↑ **76 Vulval and perineal chancre.**

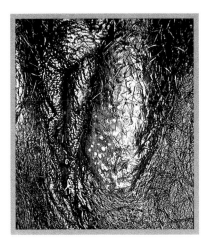

↑ **77 Labial chancre.**

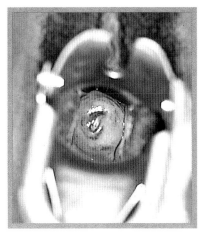

↑ **78 Early chancre of cervix**
Note similarity to cervical erosions.

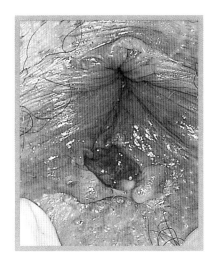

↑ **79 Primary chancre of anus.**

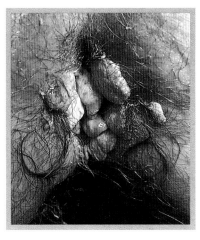

↑ **80 Primary syphilis**
Ulceration on pre-existing anal warts.

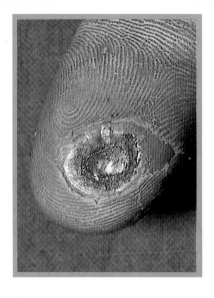

↑ **81 Primary chancre of finger.**

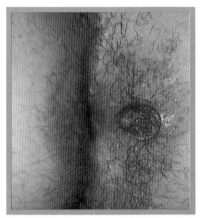

↑ **82 Buttock chancre.**

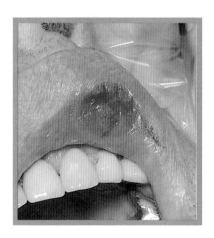

↑ **83 Lip chancre.**

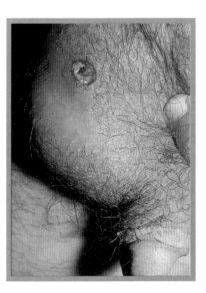

↑ **84 Scrotal chancre.**

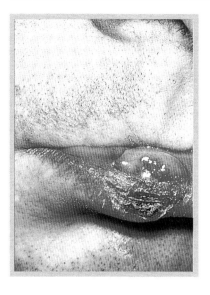

↑ 85 Primary chancre of lip.

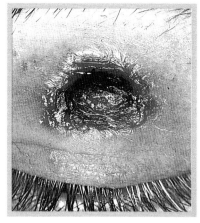

↑ 86 Primary chancre of eyelid.

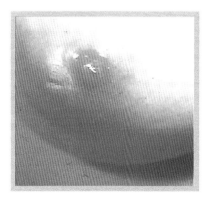

↑ 87 Primary chancre of breast.
Transmitted from an oral mucous patch.

Secondary syphilis

In secondary syphilis, the spirochaetaemia which has resulted in widespread dissemination of the organism throughout the body becomes manifest. Lesions may be found on the skin from the scalp to the soles of the feet; lesions may be found on the mucous membranes; there is often generalized lymphadenopathy and mild constitutional symptoms are common. Rarely, visceral involvement may occur. The diagram (**88**) shows the features of secondary syphilis. In about 30% of patients seen, the primary chancre is found to be present; other patients may give a history suggestive of the primary stage, but often such history is lacking.

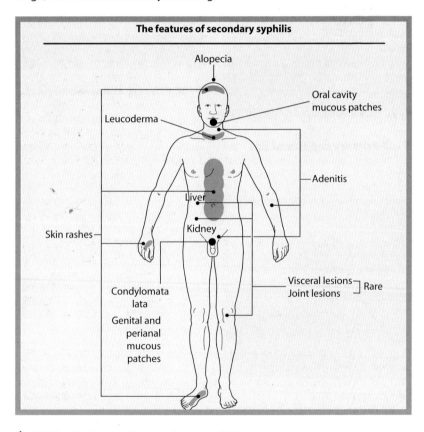

↑ **88 The features of secondary syphilis.**

Time of appearance
Signs of secondary syphilis usually appear 6–8 eight weeks after infection. Signs may appear as early as 4 weeks or, in exceptional cases, may not appear for 2 years.

Clinical presentation
With such a wide range of symptoms and signs, the permutations are almost endless. In practice, about 70% of patients with secondary syphilis first attend with a **skin rash**. Other relatively common presentations are **ulcerated lesions of the mucous membranes** or **lymph gland enlargement**. Rarer presentations include falling hair, persistent hoarseness, bone pain, hepatitis and deafness. A considerable proportion (about 30%) of patients who are found to have secondary syphilis attend at the instigation of a sexual contact. Such patients may have been aware of abnormal symptoms or signs but unaware of their significance. The generally mild constitutional symptoms are seldom a sole cause of attendance and are mentioned only when the history is taken. Many of the lesions of secondary syphilis are virtually asymptomatic and are found only in the course of comprehensive and careful examination.

After treatment, lesions usually heal quickly. Skin eruptions, if they have not been secondarily infected, disappear without residual scarring in most cases but sometimes depigmented areas may remain. Such depigmented lesions are most often seen on the neck (leukoderma). Lymphadenopathy often takes several months to resolve.

Diagnosis
The most important diagnostic method is demonstration of *T. pallidum.* Specimens for dark-ground microscopy (see p. 49) may be taken from lesions of the mucous membranes, from condylomata lata, by gland puncture (see p. 48) and occasionally from skin lesions. Serological examination is essential: practically every case of secondary syphilis shows strongly positive reactions.

It is inadequate to make the diagnosis of secondary syphilis on clinical grounds alone — the range of differential diagnosis is extremely wide. Erroneous diagnosis may result in the unnecessary and stressful attendance of sexual contacts.

Skin eruptions
Skin eruptions in secondary syphilis are characteristically **pleomorphic**, **symmetrical** and **generalized**. It is rare for the rash to be painful, pruritic or vesicular. The lesions are commonly hyperpigmented, the colour varying from pink in the early stages to a dull coppery-red in later stages. Hypopigmented lesions (leukoderma) are occasionally seen. The rash may sometimes be seen most easily when the patient has been undressed for a few minutes, i.e. when the skin is cool.

Skin rashes usually first appear as **roseolar** or **macular** eruptions; later **papular** lesions are found. Intermediate (**maculopapular**) and mixed rashes are common. Superficial scaling over papular lesions is often seen; the lesion is known as the **papulosquamous** syphilide. Particular patterns of eruption have been given descriptive topographical names in the past, e.g. annular syphilide, rupial syphilide, corymbose syphilide: these terms are now rarely used. The extremely toxic **pustular** or **malignant** syphilide, characterized by central necrosis of papular lesions, is now very rare in developed countries.

Eruptions in secondary syphilis may be very faint and with few lesions present: recognition can be extremely difficult. In non-white patients, hypertrophic lesions are more common, but often the rash is almost invisible. When the eruption is present on the scalp, patchy ('moth-eaten') alopecia may ensue.

Macular and roseolar eruptions are found mainly on the shoulder, chest, back, abdomen, buttocks, and flexor surfaces of the limbs. The macules are round or oval and 5–10 mm in diameter, although sometimes larger lesions are seen which result from coalescence of adjacent macules. The intensity of colour of the rash is very variable; it may be necessary for the patient to be undressed for several minutes before the rash can be appreciated. In one recent case, the rash was visible only after alcohol had been imbibed.

Maculopapular and papulosquamous eruptions are the most frequent and characteristic secondary syphilitic eruption.

The later lesions of cutaneous secondary syphilis show a continuous progression from the predominantly macular lesion to the predominantly squamous lesion. Initially, macular lesions develop a central induration to form a palpable nodule; superficial scaling over the papule may occur later. Papules may arise at the sites of macular lesions or may appear on previously uninvolved areas of the skin. Papular eruptions are frequently seen on the face (especially near the hair line: the 'corona veneris') and on the palms of the hands and soles of the feet. The lesions on the palms and soles are often papulosquamous in appearance. Papulosquamous lesions may occasionally be seen in other areas, usually those that are subject to friction. Tiny papular lesions occur at the mouths of hair follicles on the scalp, eyebrows, beard area and hairy areas of the trunk. This lesion is known as the **follicular syphilide**; often the atypical and misleading symptom of pruritus will be present. Papular lesions at the corner of the mouth and the nasolabial junction are often hypertrophied and 'split'. The size of papular lesions may vary from 1–15 mm in diameter; most commonly the size is between 5–10 mm.

Pustular eruptions are now rare in developed countries. This type of rash is seen most frequently in black patients and is often associated with debilitation and poor socioeconomic conditions. A few pustular lesions are quite often seen in widespread maculopapular eruptions.

Pustular lesions begin as large papules which undergo central necrosis. Severe tissue destruction and toxaemia occur and considerable scarring is likely. On the face, pustular syphilides are often extensively crusted; this lesion is known as the **rupial syphilide**.

Malignant syphilis, now almost historical, was a particularly severe form of ulcerated pustular syphilide. It has been seen recently in patients who also have HIV (see **508** and **509**).

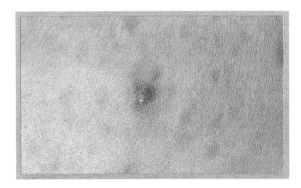

← **89 Secondary syphilis**
Macular rash (and one papular lesion).

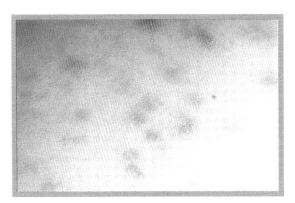

← **90 Secondary syphilis**
Maculopapular syphilide.

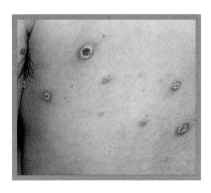

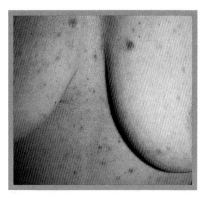

↑ 91 Secondary syphilis
Papulosquamous syphilide. Compare with Kaposi's sarcoma (**557**).

↑ 92 Secondary syphilis
Rash of chest.

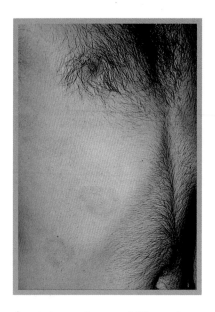

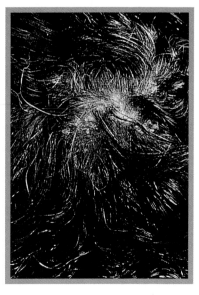

↑ 93 Secondary syphilis
Corymbose macular syphilide.

↑ 94 Secondary syphilis
Patchy alopecia ('moth-eaten scalp').

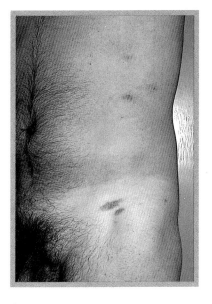

↑ 95 Secondary syphilis.

↑ 96 Secondary syphilis
Same patient as **95**.

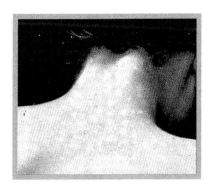

↑ 97 Secondary syphilis
Patchy depigmentation of neck
(leukoderma, colli venus) and upper
back, residual after treatment.

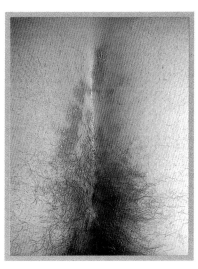

↑ 98 Secondary syphilis
Natal cleft.

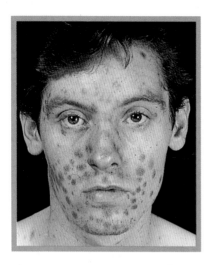

↑ 99 Secondary syphilis
Typical papular syphilide of face. Note perioral distribution.

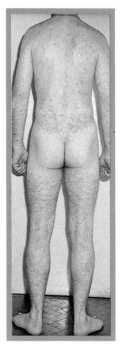

← 100 Secondary syphilis Maculo-papular rash.

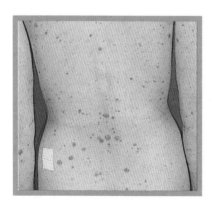

↑ 101 Secondary syphilis
Papulosquamous syphilide: the adhesive plaster marks the site of skin biopsy.

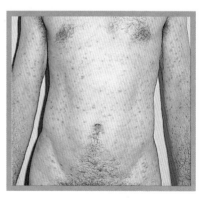

↑ 102 Secondary syphilide
Maculopapular rash.

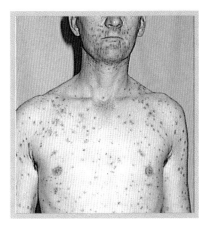

← 103 Secondary syphilis
Very typical papulosquamous syphilide. Note the facial lesions, the colour and the symmetrical distribution. This rash had been present for 3 months before diagnosis and only cleared completely 6 months after completion of treatment.

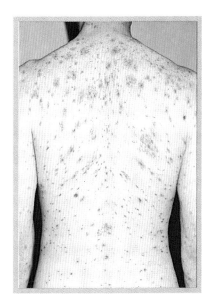

↑ 104 Secondary syphilis
Back of patient shown in **103**. Note the distribution of the rash, reminiscent of pityriasis rosea (**400**).

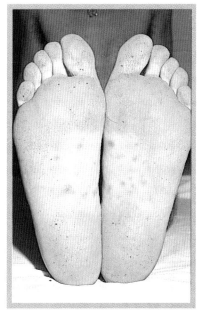

↑ 105 Secondary syphilis
Plantar lesions.

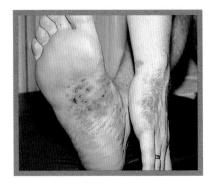

← 106 Secondary syphilis
Carpal and plantar syphilide.

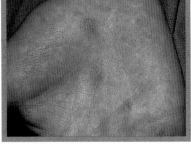

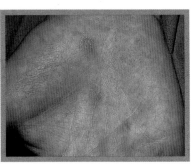

↑ 107 Secondary syphilis
Palmar lesions.

↑ 108 Secondary syphilis
Mucous patches on penis and
scrotum.

Condylomata lata

Condylomata lata are modified papular lesions found at anatomical sites where friction and moisture are present: they occur concurrently with the skin eruption. Condylomata lata are most frequently found around the anus and vulva. Lesions may also occur on the penis, scrotum, thigh, axilla, angle of the mouth and beneath a pendulous breast. The lesions are pale brown or pale pinky-grey in colour, 5–20 mm in diameter. Initially, the lesions are discrete and circular but coalescence may occur to form a large lesion with a polycyclic outline. The surface of the lesion is slightly raised, flat and clean, and is usually moist from exuded serum. Microscopically, this serum swarms with *T. pallidum*. Condylomata lata are the most highly infectious lesions in syphilis.

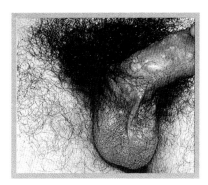

↑ **109 Secondary syphilis**
Condylomata lata on penis and
scrotum, maculopapular rash on thigh.

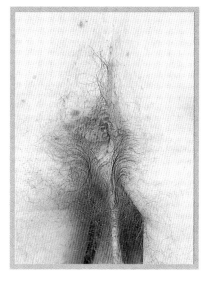

↑ **110 Secondary syphilis**
Perianal mucous patches and
maculopapular syphilide.

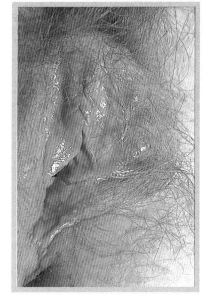

↑ **111 Condylomata lata of
vulva.**

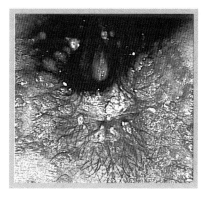

↑ **112 Condylomata lata of
vulva and anus.**

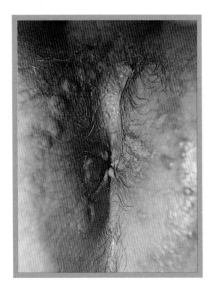

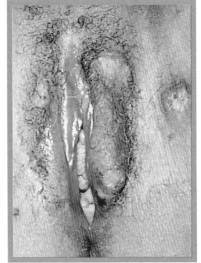

↑ **113 Condylomata lata**
Perianal. Note resemblance to warts.

↑ **114 Secondary syphilis**
Condylomata lata of vulva.

Lesions of mucous membranes

Lesions of the mucous membranes occur concurrently with the cutaneous eruptions in secondary syphilis. The lesions are termed **mucous patches**. Mucous patches are most commonly seen on the inner surface of the lips but are also found on other oral mucous membranes (including the tongue), in the pharynx and on the larynx. In the latter situation, the lesion may cause hoarseness but the mucous patches are difficult to see without laryngoscopy. **Genital mucous membranes** may also be involved. In male patients, mucous patches are found beneath the prepuce and on the glans penis; in female patients, the lesions occur on the mucosal surfaces of the labia and vulva and, rarely, on the vaginal wall and cervix. All these lesions are highly infectious.

Mucous patches are round, oval or serpiginous (**'snail-track ulcer'**) in outline. The lesion is usually a superficial erosion but occasionally papules are seen. The mucous patch may be dull red in colour or covered with an easily removed grey membrane; the margin of the lesion is marked by an erythematous areola. On the surface of the tongue, mucous patches look like bald areas: the appearance results from destruction of the filiform papillae.

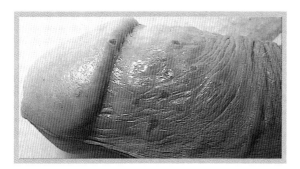

← 115 Secondary syphilis
Mucous patches of prepuce. Note resemblance to herpes genitalis (cf. **300**).

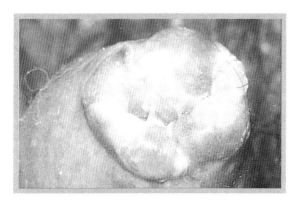

← 116 Secondary syphilis
Mucous patches of prepuce (cf. **67**, **355**).

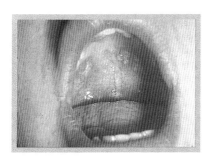

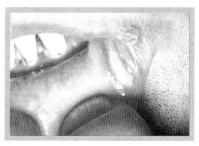

↑ 117 Secondary syphilis
Vesicopapular lesions and 'snail-track' ulcers of hard palate.

↑ 118 Secondary syphilis
Mucous patch of upper lip with typical adherent exudate.

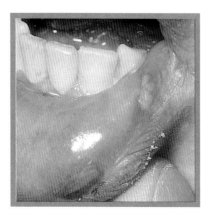

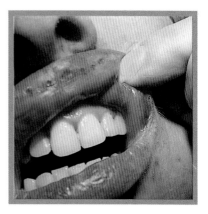

↑ 119 Secondary syphilis
Mucous patch of lower lip. Note
resemblance to Behçet's syndrome
(**367**).

↑ 120 Secondary syphilis
Mucous patches of upper lip:
compare with erythema multiforme
(**491**).

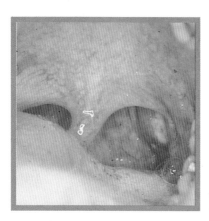

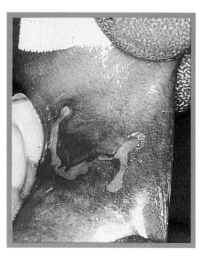

↑ 121 Secondary syphilis
Mucous patch of fauces: this lesion
may be a primary chancre.
Corymbose skin lesions from the
same patient are shown in **93**.

↑ 122 Secondary syphilis
'Snail-track' ulcer on lip.

Latent syphilis

The stage in the progress of the infection known as **latent syphilis** begins when the superficial lesions and other manifestations of secondary syphilis resolve. The patient with latent syphilis has no outward signs of infection, but positive serological tests (and sometimes changes in the cerebrospinal fluid (CSF)) indicate the disease. Latent syphilis may persist for the rest of the patient's life, but traditionally about 40% of untreated latent syphilitics develop **tertiary syphilis**. Our own experience suggests that the traditional ratio of 6 latent syphilis: 4 tertiary syphilis is no longer correct and that the ratio at present is nearer 20:1. The reason for this change may be that, in the course of a lifetime, many individuals with unrecognized syphilis receive for other conditions antibiotic therapy which is coincidentally treponemicidal and which halts progression of the syphilitic infection. **Investigation of sexual contacts and children should always be considered.**

Tertiary syphilis

At present, most patients found to have tertiary syphilis with the classical syndromes of **aortic regurgitation** and **aneurysm**, **tabes** and **general paralysis of the insane** will have initially attended and been diagnosed in other medical departments: they are later referred to the STD clinic. Initial attendance of a patient with tertiary syphilis at an STD clinic is therefore rare; for this reason a full account of the protean manifestations of tertiary syphilis is not given here. For fuller information, readers are referred to comprehensive textbooks.

The basic pathological lesion in tertiary syphilis is a chronic granuloma known as a **gumma**. The gumma is an area of tissue necrosis, resulting from ischaemia caused by endarteritis, surrounded by granulation tissue. It is a slowly progressive lesion; in most clinical cases, areas of activity and regression can be recognized. The individual gumma may vary in size from 2–30 mm; often multiple lesions (gummata) are present. A diffuse fibrotic form of gummatous infiltration is occasionally seen.

The traditional figures show:

Approximately 15%: involvement of the skin, subcutaneous tissues, bones and periosteal tissues (**'benign late syphilis'**). Occurs 3–20 years after initial infection. Relatively more common in black patients.

Approximately 12%: involvement of the heart and/or aorta and (rarely) other parts of the cardiovascular system. Occurs 10–30 years after initial infection. Relatively more common in males and blacks.

Approximately 12%: involvement of the nervous system. The lesions may be meningeal, vascular or parenchymatous; mixed forms are common. Occurs 3–7 years (meningovascular) and 10–20 years (parenchymatous) after initial infection.

Other forms of tertiary syphilis are rare, although gummata have been described in practically every named anatomical structure. Some patients with no clinical abnormalities are found to have abnormal CSF findings (asymptomatic neurosyphilis); the prognostic significance of this finding is not clear. Occasionally paroxysmal haemoglobinuria may occur in late syphilis as a result of the presence of a circulating haemolysin. **Investigation of sexual contacts and children should always be considered.**

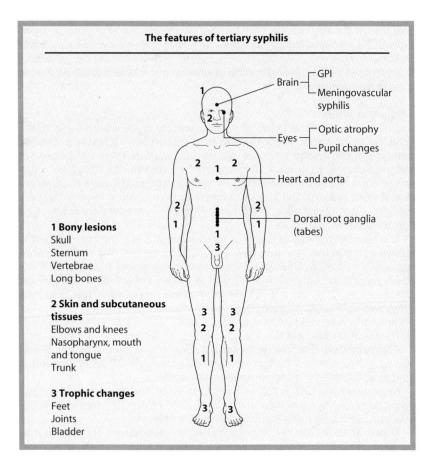

The features of tertiary syphilis

Brain — GPI / Meningovascular syphilis

Eyes — Optic atrophy / Pupil changes

Heart and aorta

Dorsal root ganglia (tabes)

1 Bony lesions
Skull
Sternum
Vertebrae
Long bones

2 Skin and subcutaneous tissues
Elbows and knees
Nasopharynx, mouth and tongue
Trunk

3 Trophic changes
Feet
Joints
Bladder

↑ **123 The features of tertiary syphilis.**

Skin lesions

Nodulocutaneous syphilides. Nodules, single or grouped, appear in the skin and slowly increase in size. The whole lesion may be extensive, but individual nodules seldom exceed 1 cm in diameter. The lesion may remain nodular or, more commonly, ulcerates. Most lesions show evidence of simultaneous activity and regression, with ulceration at the periphery and healing at the centre of the involved area. The ulcer is **'punched-out'** and is circular (or polycyclic) in outline; groups of lesions may show annular, gyrate or serpiginous topography. There is often an adherent basal slough, termed **'wash-leather slough'**. Squamous change (scaling) may overlie non-ulcerated nodules occurring on the palms and soles. After treatment or spontaneous healing, characteristic non-contractile **'tissue-paper'** scarring persists, often showing areas of hypo- or hyperpigmentation.

Gummatous ulcers are painless and may cause severe tissue destruction before the patient seeks advice. They are most frequently found on the face, trunk and thigh but no region is exempt.

Subcutaneous gummata. These gummata originate as subcutaneous or deeper (e.g. periosteal) nodules which become attached to, and later ulcerate through, the skin. The lesions are usually single and may be up to 4–5 cm in diameter. The clinical appearance and location is similar to the nodulocutaneous syphilides. Severe and deep tissue destruction may occur.

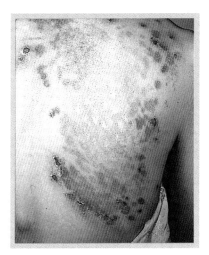

← 124 Tertiary syphilis
Nodulocutaneous syphilide of back with hyperpigmented scarring.

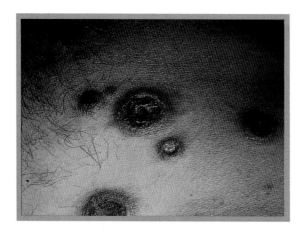

← 125 Tertiary syphilis
Multiple gummatous ulcers of chest wall.

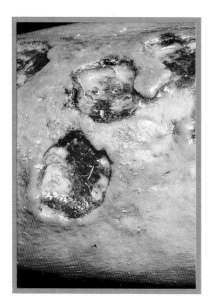

↑ 126 Tertiary syphilis
Typical gummatous ulcers, showing vertical margins and 'wash-leather' slough.

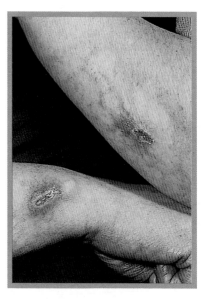

↑ 127 Tertiary syphilis
Hypopigmented 'tissue-paper' scarring at sites of healed gummatous ulcers.

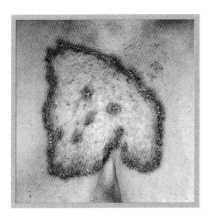

↑ **128 Tertiary syphilis**
Nodulocutaneous ulceration of chest wall, showing peripheral activity, central healing and hypopigmentation.

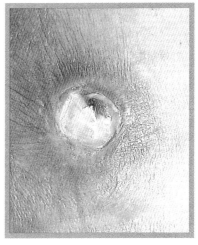

↑ **129 Tertiary syphilis**
Gumma of ankle.

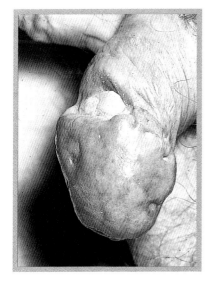

← **130 Tertiary syphilis**
Gumma of penis.

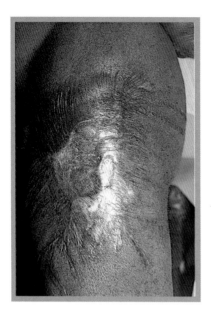

↑ 131 Tertiary syphilis
'Tissue-paper' scarring over healed gumma of hip.

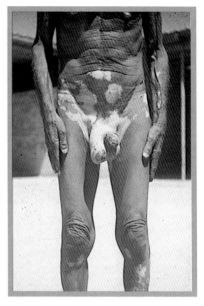

↑ 132 Tertiary syphilis
Hypopigmentation following healing of extensive gummatous ulceration. Compare with **161** (late pinta).

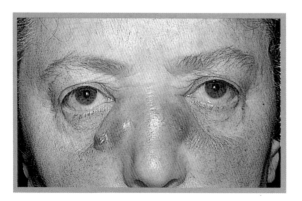

← 133 Tertiary syphilis
Periosteal gummata of nasal bones.

Cardiovascular lesions

It is not appropriate in this book to describe in detail late syphilis of the cardiovascular system. Patients with these conditions are rare and usually present at cardiac, thoracic or vascular clinics. The classical syndromes are :

· Aortic regurgitation
· Aneurysm of the ascending aorta
· Coronary ostial stenosis.

Mixed forms are frequently encountered.

Syphilitic aortitis precedes the development of the recognizable syndromes but probably cannot be diagnosed *ante mortem*. Occasionally, syphilitic involvement of other arteries may occur. About 30% of patients with cardiovascular syphilis also have symptomatic or asymptomatic neurosyphilis. Examination must always include neurological assessment and lumbar puncture.

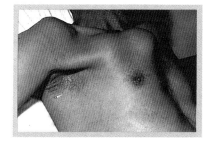

↑ 134 Tertiary syphilis
Aneurysm of ascending aorta which has eroded the sternum and extended on to the chest wall.

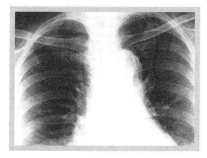

↑ 135 Tertiary syphilis
X-ray of aortic aneurysm Note linear calcification in aortic wall.

Neurosyphilis

As with cardiovascular syphilis, it has not been thought appropriate to describe the now rare syndromes of neurosyphilis in detail. The classical syndromes are :

• **General paralysis of the insane (GPI)**
• **Tabes dorsalis (locomotor ataxia)**.

Mixed forms are common (**taboparesis**).

The meninges and vascular supply of the brain and spinal cord may be involved; occasionally **primary optic atrophy** may be the sole abnormality in neurosyphilis. **Asymptomatic neurosyphilis** (abnormal CSF findings with normal neurological examination) is nearly as frequent as **symptomatic** neurosyphilis. Cardiovascular syphilis may coexist with neurological involvement. Complete examination must include clinical and radiological assessment of the heart and aorta.

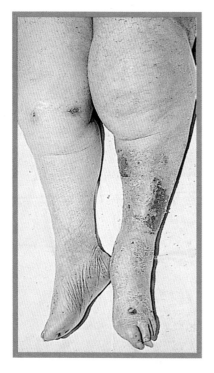

← 136 Tertiary syphilis
Charcot arthropathy of knees: tabes dorsalis.

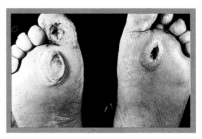

↑ 137 Tertiary syphilis
Perforating ulcers of foot in tabes dorsalis.

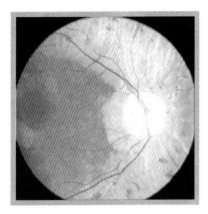

↑ **138 Tertiary syphilis**
Pale optic disc with 'bone spicule' pigmentation. Both late-stage findings in a retina affected by syphilis.

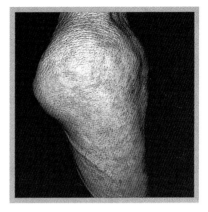

↑ **139 Tertiary syphilis**
Charcot arthropathy of elbow: tabes dorsalis.

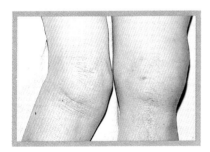

← **140 Tertiary syphilis**
 Charcot arthropathy of knees: tabes dorsalis. Note the hypermobility of the joint.

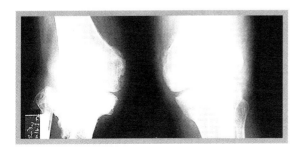

← **141 Tertiary syphilis**
X-ray of **140**.

Bone lesions

Tertiary syphilis of the bones generally begins as a **periostitis**, with later cortical involvement. The **osteoperiostitis** of long bones is predominantly an osteoblastic process (there is usually radiological evidence of adjacent osteoclastosis) with deposition of extra bone under the periosteum, resulting in the usual clinical findings of thickening and irregularity of affected areas. Syphilitic osteoperiostitis of the bones of the skull and nasal skeleton is predominantly osteoclastic, giving the clinical finding of bone loss, which occasionally is very extensive.

About 50% of patients with tertiary syphilis of bone complain of pain in affected areas; this pain may be very severe and is classically described as 'boring' in character; even after antisyphilitic treatment, the pain may persist for a long time. Tenderness of the affected areas is often found. Radiological survey of patients with symptomatic bony syphilis often discloses further areas of asymptomatic involvement. Pathological fractures may occur and are sometimes the presenting symptom.

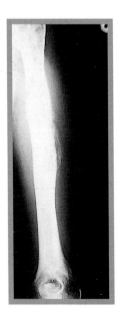

↑ **142 Tertiary syphilis**
X-ray of osteitis of humerus.

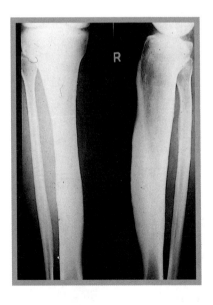

↑ **143 Tertiary syphilis**
X-ray of periostitis of tibia. Compare with 'sabre' tibia in yaws, **172**.

Oral cavity lesions

The oral and nasal cavities are commonly involved in tertiary syphilis. Gummatous ulceration may be found on any of the mucous membranes. Diffuse gummatous infiltration of the tongue may result in chronic superficial or interstitial glossitis: rarely, diffuse infiltration may involve the lips. Syphilitic osteitis and periostitis may involve the bones of the nose or palate; palatal perforation and destruction, sometimes gross, of the nasal skeleton may be found.

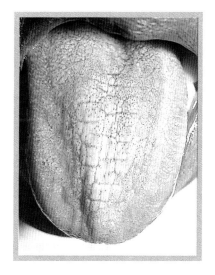

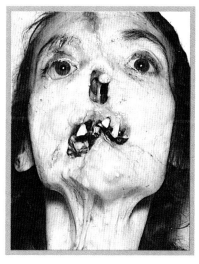

↑ **144 Tertiary syphilis**
Chronic interstitial glossitis. This lesion was completely asymptomatic and persisted after treatment.

↑ **145 Tertiary syphilis**
Gross gummatous destruction of face. Compare with **155** (endemic syphilis) and **175** (yaws).

Congenital syphilis

In untreated syphilis it is thought that waves of spirochaetaemia occur, diminishing in frequency as time passes. Transmission of syphilis to the fetus occurs when pregnancy coincides with spirochaetaemia. The observed great variation in severity of congenital syphilis is probably dependent on the degree of spirochaetaemia at the time the fetus is initially infected.

In acquired syphilis, the portal of entry of infection is the site of the primary chancre; in congenital syphilis, *T. pallidum* enters the circulation directly through the placental capillaries. The clinical manifestations correspond to the secondary and later stages of acquired syphilis.

Congenital syphilis is a rarity in developed countries, where antenatal care includes serological tests for syphilis so that infected mothers are treated before delivery. In these circumstances, active congenital syphilis is almost unknown, but children infected *in utero* may sometimes show clinical evidence of the effects of the infection present before treatment was begun (e.g. Hutchinson's teeth).

Detailed consideration of congenital syphilis is given in the standard textbooks. In this book, only a few representative pictures of clinical manifestations are included. **It is very important to remember that a diagnosis of congenital syphilis is the starting point for a complete family investigation.**

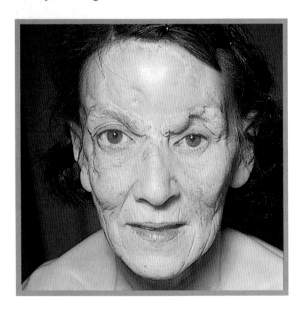

← **146 Congenital syphilis**
Scarring resulting from extensive gummata.

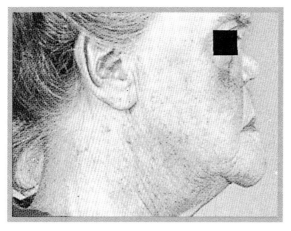

← 147 Congenital syphilis
Profile of facies. Note the depressed bridge (flat profile) of the nose.

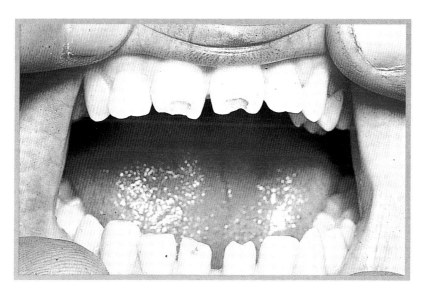

↑ 148 Congenital syphilis
Hutchinson's incisors: the 'screwdriver' shape with marginal notching and distal narrowing.

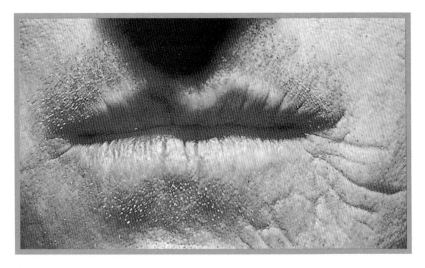

↑ 149 Congenital syphilis
Perioral rhagades, scarring from healed perioral lesions. Similar lesions are sometimes seen in the perianal region.

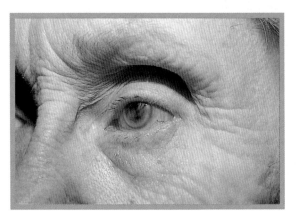

← 150 Congenital syphilis
Faint corneal nebulae resulting from previous interstitial keratitis.

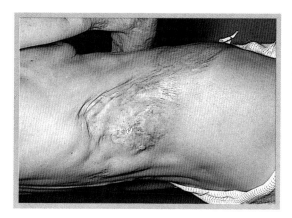

← 151 Congenital syphilis
Extensive scarring from previous gummata: same patient as **146**.

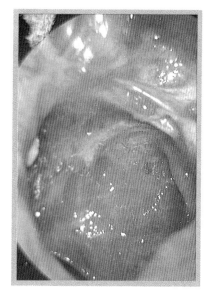

← 152 Congenital syphilis
Large perforation of hard palate.

NON-VENEREAL TREPONEMATOSES
Endemic syphilis

Endemic syphilis is the non-venereal form of the disease. Most infections are acquired in childhood with subsequent diminished susceptibility to sexually transmitted treponematosis in adult life. It is a disease found in communities with low socioeconomic status and was formerly widespread. With rising standards of nutrition, clothing and hygiene, the incidence of endemic syphilis declines; at present, foci of infection are still to be found in some areas of Africa and the Middle East. Endemic syphilis is essentially the same disease throughout the world, but each area has its own local name for the disease. Extant names include *bejel* (Iraq) and *njovera* (Zimbabwe) *inter alia*; historical names include the 'button scurvy' (Ireland) and *skerljevo* (Balkan countries).

The infectious stages of the disease are mainly seen in children, as the disease is spread by direct contact (usually from other children), or by shared objects such as drinking or eating utensils and, possibly, by insect vectors.

Clinically, the disease resembles venereal syphilis, but primary lesions are rarely identified. Many patients present with moist lesions of the oral mucous membranes or condylomata lata, or may be found to have latent infection or skin or bone gummata. Cardiovascular and neurological involvement seem to be rare. Congenital transmission is also rare as untreated females are generally non-infectious when the fertile years are reached; conversely, an infant infected from another source may superinfect the parent.

Treponema pallidum seen in lesions of endemic syphilis is indistinguishable from the organism seen in venereal syphilis. The distinction between the two forms of the disease is not absolute but depends on the consideration of clinical and epidemiological factors.

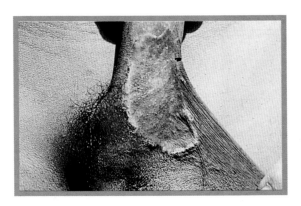

← **153 Early endemic syphilis**
Annular rash on penis of a Zimbabwean patient.

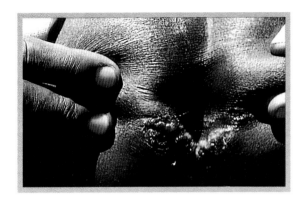

← 154 Early endemic syphilis
Anal papillomata: compare with condylomata lata (**113**) and yaws (**170**).

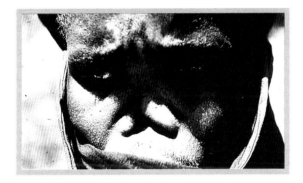

← 155 Late endemic syphilis
Gangosa (gummatous destruction of the face). Compare with **147** (congenital syphilis) and **175** (yaws).

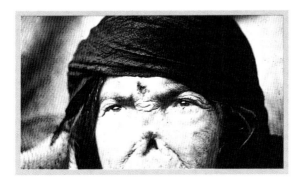

← 156 Late endemic syphilis
Destruction caused by nasal gummata in bejel.

Pinta (mal de pinto, carate)

Pinta is the least serious of the treponematoses. The disease has a limited distribution (see map) and is almost confined to economically disadvantaged indigenous and black communities. Transmission is by contagion and nearly always occurs before adult life.

The clinical lesions are known as **pintides**. The **primary pintide** appears, usually on exposed skin surfaces, after an average incubation period of 6–8 weeks. The lesion is circular, erythematous and desquamating, with a diameter of 1–2 cm. **Secondary pintides** appear several months later. These are of similar form and may be adjacent to the primary lesion or disseminated. Hyperpigmentation of secondary lesions is common; their colour may be reddish, bluish or black. **Tertiary pintides** appear after a latent period of some years; dyschromia is usual, with late lesions often completely depigmented. Hyperkeratosis may occur in secondary and tertiary stages and is particularly common with pintides on the palms or soles. Visceral involvement and congenital transmission (if they occur at all) are extremely rare.

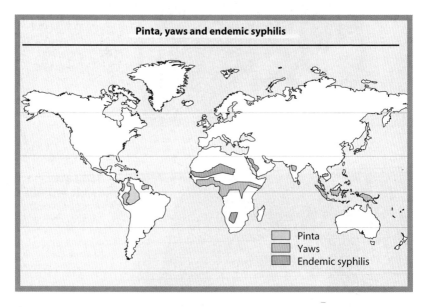

↑ **157 Pinta, yaws and endemic syphilis**
Distribution.

The causative organism is *Treponema carateum*: it may be recognized in dark-ground specimens taken from primary and secondary pintides. *Treponema carateum* is morphologically identical to *T. pallidum*. Serological tests for syphilis give positive results in pinta, indistinguishable from the results obtained in venereal syphilis.

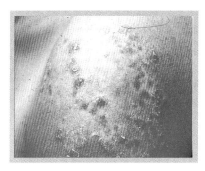

← 158 Pinta
Early pintide. Note the similarity to maculopapular syphilides (**90**).

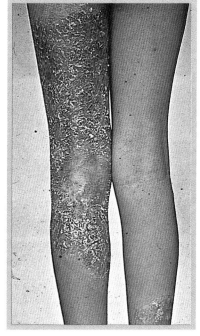

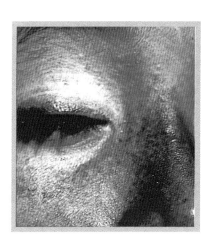

↑ 159 Pinta
Pintide of nose and cheek showing typical slate-blue pigmentation.

↑ 160 Pinta
Late pintide of leg, hyperpigmented lesions.

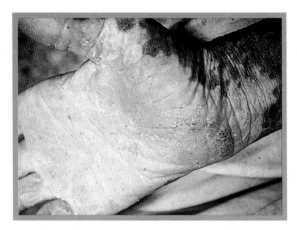

← 161 Pinta
Late pintide, 'glove hand' showing achromia.

Yaws (pian, framboesia)

Yaws, the non-venereal treponematosis of tropical regions, was formerly extremely common. Mass treatment campaigns by the World Health Organization (WHO) have greatly reduced the incidence. Transmission of the disease is by contagion and occurs in most cases in childhood. The pattern of the disease is broadly similar to syphilis, as primary, secondary, latent and tertiary stages occur, and clinical lesions show considerable similarity. As in the other non-venereal treponemal diseases, cardiovascular and neurological involvement and congenital transmission are thought to be very rare.

The **primary lesion (mother yaw)** may be found anywhere on the skin, but is usually on an exposed surface such as the lower part of the leg. The lesion is initially a papule which enlarges to an exuberant granuloma with papillomatous margins, 2–6 cm in diameter. Local lymph gland enlargement is common. The mother yaw is often secondarily infected with pyogenic organisms so that residual scarring is frequent.

In **secondary yaws**, skin eruptions similar to those seen in secondary syphilis occur; these are often hypertrophic. The most characteristic eruption is the papillomatous rash—**framboesiomata**. The multiple red (or yellow crusted) papillomata, 5–20 mm in diameter, are found mainly at mucocutaneous junctions and on other moist surfaces of the body, but may occur on any skin surface. Painful papillomata and hyperkeratosis may occur on the soles: the term '**crab yaws**' has been applied to these painful lesions which cause the patient to walk with a crab-like gait. Generalized lymph gland enlargement is often found. Painful areas of osteitis and periostitis may occur: dactylitis is seen in children; characteristic broadening of the bridge of the nose caused by maxillary periostitis is known as **goundou**.

In **tertiary yaws**, skin lesions similar to nodulocutaneous syphilides and gummatous ulcers occur and may later heal with extensive scarring and hypopigmentation. Painful bone lesions are often found, particularly affecting the long bones. The characteristic lesion is the '**sabre tibia**'. Extensive bone and soft-tissue involvement of the face sometimes occurs; the condition is known as **gangosa** and may result in gross deformity. Juxta-articular nodes are another characteristic lesion of late yaws.

The causative organism, *Treponema pertenue*, can be found in dark-ground preparations taken in the primary and secondary stages from skin lesions and enlarged glands. It is morphologically identical to *Treponema pallidum*. The serological tests for syphilis give positive results in yaws. A recurrent problem is the evaluation of positive serological tests for syphilis in clinically normal patients who originate in yaws-endemic areas: a definite diagnosis is usually impossible to establish (see p. 61).

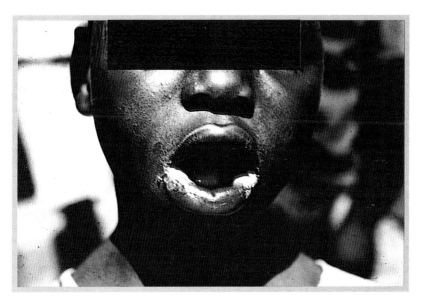

↑ **162 Early yaws**
Lip lesions.

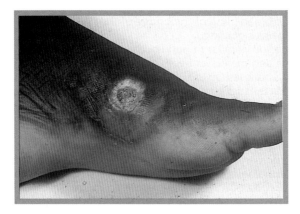

← 163 Primary yaws
Compare with primary syphilis, **63** and **84**.

← 164 Secondary yaws
Hypertrophic papulosquamous skin lesions.

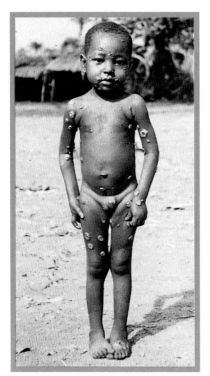

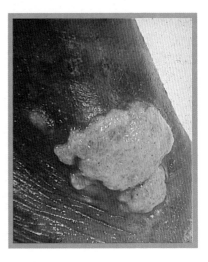

↑ 165 Secondary yaws
Framboesioma.

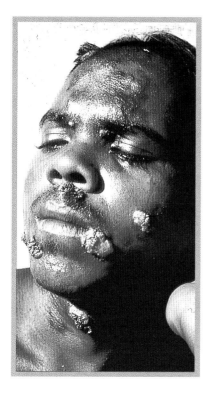

← 166 Secondary yaws
Facial papillomata.

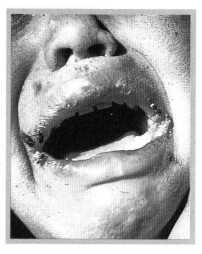

↑ 167 Secondary yaws
Split papule at corner of mouth. Note
flies, possible vectors of infection.

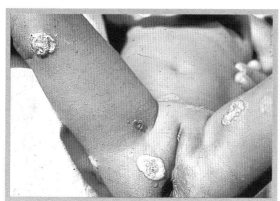

**← 168 Secondary
yaws**
Condylomata and
papillomata.

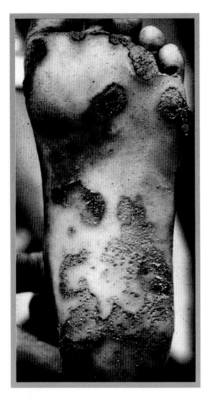

← 169 Secondary yaws
'Crab yaws' of foot: note 'worm-eaten' appearance.

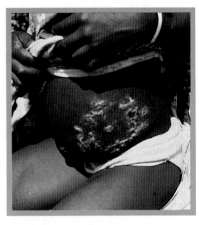

↑170 Secondary yaws
Corymbose lesions. Compare with **131,** healed syphilitic gumma.

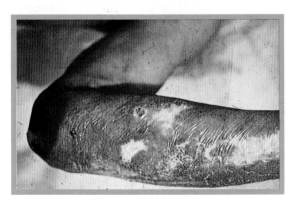

←171 Late yaws
Gummata of arm.
Compare with **151**.

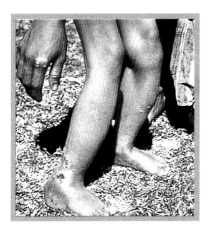

↑172 Late yaws
'Sabre' tibiae, a very typical lesion.
(The hand belongs to a nurse).

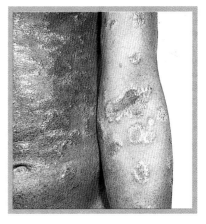

↑ 173 Late yaws
Extensive gummata, shown shortly
after treatment was started (cf. **153**).

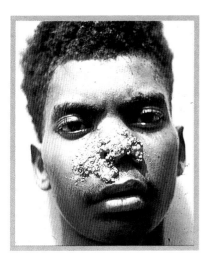

↑ 174 Late yaws
Early gangosa.

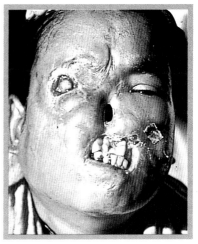

↑ 175 Late yaws
Late gangosa.

CHANCROID, DONOVANOSIS AND LYMPHOGRANULOMA VENEREUM (LGV)

CHANCROID (SOFT SORE, ULCUS MOLLE, SOFT CHANCRE)

Chancroid is an acute sexually transmitted infection of the genitalia characterized by painful ulceration and frequent bubo formation. It is found throughout the world but is much more frequently seen in warm climates and in populations with low standards of hygiene. In Western Europe and North America, the disease is now rare. Chancroid is highly infectious, but clinical lesions are disproportionately rare in women, suggesting that a 'carrier' state occurs although recent research suggests this is uncommon.

Cause

The causative organism is a bacterium, *Haemophilus ducreyi*.

Clinical course

The incubation period averages 3–6 days, but shorter and longer periods have been reported occasionally. The clinical lesion begins as a painful vesicular papule, which rapidly progresses to an ulcer with a bright red areola and shelving margins. The ulcer may be round or irregular in outline; adjacent lesions often become confluent. Secondary infection is common and considerable tissue destruction may ensue. Lesions may be single or multiple, with a diameter ranging from 3–20 mm. Chancroidal ulcers may be found anywhere on the genitals, but are most frequent at the sites where trauma during intercourse is most likely. In males, these sites are at the preputial margin or on the coronal sulcus and fraenum, and in females on the labia and perineum. Occasionally extragenital lesions are found, usually caused by autoinoculation from adjacent genital ulcers.

Painful enlargement of the inguinal lymph nodes (**chancroidal bubo**) occurs 7–14 days later in about 50% of cases. Sometimes the patient presents with the bubo, the initial ulcer having been unnoticed. The enlarged glands may be unilateral or bilateral and usually lie above the inguinal ligament. The bubo is a mass of glands matted together and is often adherent to the overlying erythematous and oedematous skin. Central softening is often found and, untreated, the bubo may rupture and discharge through a fistula. Occasionally, extensive involvement of the skin around the fistulous opening occurs.

Diagnosis

Many cases are diagnosed on clinical grounds alone. It is important to exclude other concurrent diseases, e.g. syphilis.

Haemophilus ducreyi may be recognised in stained preparations made from the surface of the ulcer or bubo pus, but recognition is often difficult because of other organisms present. Culture is difficult and thus insensitive but specific.

110

A serological test is not available and other tests such as various nucleic acid probes are in development. Skin tests are outdated.

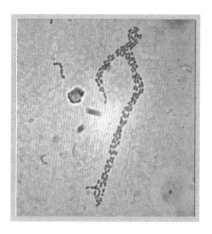

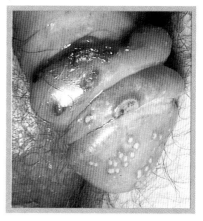

↑ **176 *Haemophilus ducreyi***
Photomicrograph showing 'school of fish' growth pattern.

↑ **177 Penile chancroid**
with secondary bacterial vesicopustules.

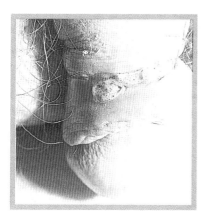

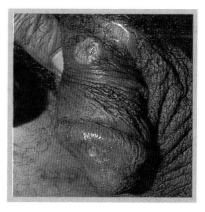

↑ **178 Chancroid**
of prepuce.

↑ **179 Chancroid**
Early ulceration.

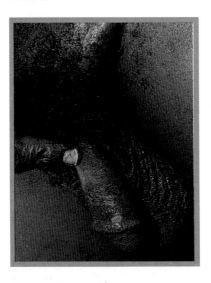

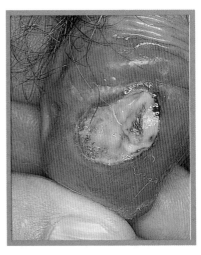

↑ **180 Chancroid**
Ulcer and bubo.

↑ **181 Typical chancroid**
of glans penis. Note considerable tissue destruction and adherent slough.

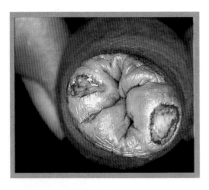

↑ **182 Chancroid**
of prepuce. Note the considerable oedema and erythematous halo. After treatment of this type of lesion phimosis may occur.

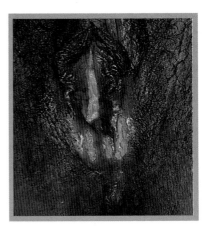

↑ **183 Chancroid**
of vulva.

DONOVANOSIS (GRANULOMA INGUINALE; GRANULOMA VENEREUM)

Donovanosis is a chronic, slowly progressive, ulcerative disease of the genitalia and adjacent tissues. It is probable that transmission is by sexual contact although this has not yet been definitely proved. Sexual consorts of patients with the disease are often apparently uninfected. The disease is most often seen in black or coloured races, and is most frequently encountered in tropical or subtropical areas. Males are more frequently affected than females.

Cause

The causative organism is an intracellular parasite, *Calymmatobacterium granulomatis*, formerly known as *Donovania granulomatosis*. The organism was first recognized in 1905.

Clinical course

The incubation period is usually between 10 and 40 days, but periods as short as 3 days and as long as 84 days have been reported.

The clinical lesion begins as a painless vesicle or indurated papule. This lesion becomes eroded to form an ulcer with a beefy red granular base. The ulcer is usually round with a rolled edge. Centrifugal spread occurs, usually eccentrically, and the advancing edge of the lesion spreads on the surface from the primary site to the adjacent tissue. Subcutaneous extension also occurs — in the inguinal region, this may be mistaken for lymph gland involvement and is known as a **pseudobubo**. Subcutaneous abscesses may occur. In the absence of treatment, healing is uncommon and the granulated area may become secondarily infected or undergo neoplastic change.

Donovanosis lesions are found initially on the shaft of the penis, the labia or the perianal region and (rarely) on the vaginal wall or cervix. Spread of the disease commonly involves the groin, perineum or natal cleft. Rarely, extragenital lesions may be found.

Diagnosis

C. granulomatis can usually be easily identified in suitably stained smears of material taken from the active edge of a lesion. Culture is possible but rarely achieved. The painless ulceration in early stages may mimic syphilis; tests to exclude syphilis are essential.

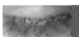
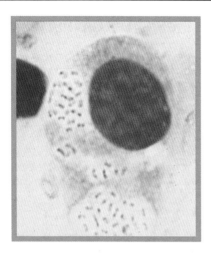

↑ 184 Photomicrograph of tissue smear showing *Calymmatobacterium granulomatis*
Note the deeper staining at the poles of the organism ('safety pin').

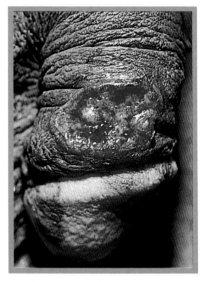

↑ 185 Granuloma inguinale
Lesion on penile shaft.

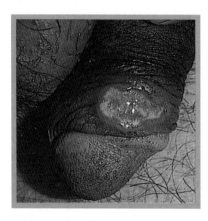

↑ 186 Donovanosis
Lesion on penile shaft showing 'rolled edge'.

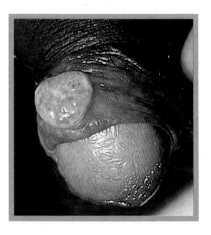

↑ 187 Donovanosis
Exuberant lesion of prepuce.

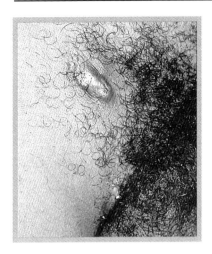

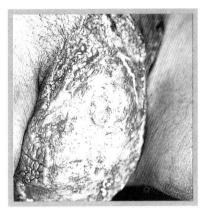

↑ **189 Late Donovanosis**
Extensive involvement of scrotum
and pathological amputation of the
penis.

↑ **188 Donovanosis**
Bubo.

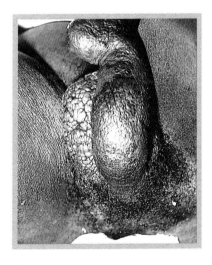

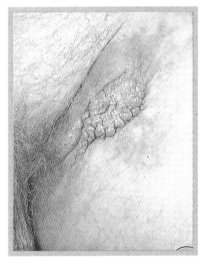

↑ **190 Late Donovanosis**
Involvement of penis and scrotum
with gross scarring and contraction.

↑ **191 Donovanosis**
of groin.

115

LYMPHOGRANULOMA VENEREUM (LYMPHOGRANULOMA INGUINALE, NICOLAS–FAVRE DISEASE, CLIMATIC BUBO)

Lymphogranuloma venereum (**LGV**) is a chronic, sexually transmitted disease whose main effects result from damage to the lymphatic system draining the site of infection. The disease is universal but is much more prevalent in tropical and subtropical areas.

Cause

The infection is caused by the LGV biovar of *Chlamydia trachomatis* (serovars L1, L2 and L3). This microorganism, an obligate intracellular parasite, is a variant of the trachoma biovar of *C. trachomatis*, which is associated with trachoma and a wide variety of oculogenital infections.

Clinical course

The incubation period is usually between 7 and 15 days, but longer and shorter periods have been reported.

The **primary stage** is a small painless papule or ulcer. It may be found anywhere on the external genitalia but is rarely recognized in women; in men, most primary lesions are seen on the shaft or corona of the penis. The lesion is transient and often unnoticed by the patient. The disease usually presents in the **secondary stage** with unilateral or bilateral enlargement of inguinal lymph nodes (**inguinal syndrome**). These enlarged glands (buboes) usually occur after the primary lesion has healed, with an average incubation period of 3–4 weeks. The enlarged glands are matted together and may occur both above and below the inguinal ligament (the **'groove sign'**). Pain in the bubo is usual; constitutional symptoms are common. Central softening and multiple fistula formation may ensue. Rectal involvement is also described in this stage in both women and homosexual males (**anorectal syndrome**).

The **late, or tertiary, stage** of the disease results from the blockage of lymphatic channels by the infection. Distal oedema develops, which may result in gross elephantiasis of the genitals. In females, the vulval elephantiasis and associated tissue destruction is known as **esthiomène**. Rectal stricture formation (and complications such as fistula development) may also occur in late LGV, more often in females .

Diagnosis

Intracellular inclusions may be recognized in stained smears of material from lesions or bubo aspirate, or by tissue culture. Serum can be tested for IgG and IgM class antibodies to the appropriate Chlamydia serovars. A rising titre of the LGV/*Psittacosis* complement fixation test is rarely seen but an elevated titre (> 1:64 in 50% of cases) is strongly supportive of the clinical diagnosis. The intradermal Frei test is insensitive, non-specific and outdated.

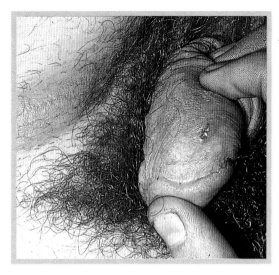

← **192
Lymphogranuloma
venereum**
Primary ulcer and groin
bubo.

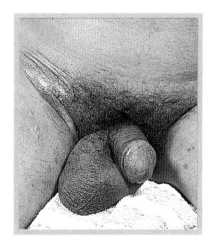

↑ **193 Lymphogranuloma
venereum**
Same patient as in **192**. The
discharging bubo is never seen in
syphilis.

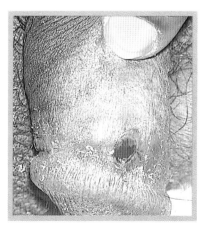

↑ **194 Lymphogranuloma
venereum (LGV)**
Primary lesion in coronal sulcus. Note
similarity to primary syphilis (**63**).

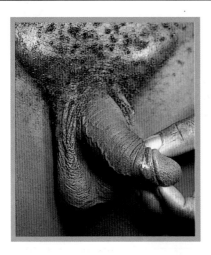

↑ 195 Lymphogranuloma venereum
Bilateral bubos.

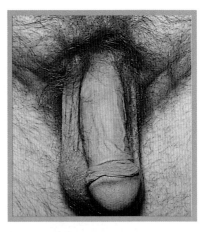

↑ 196 Bilateral lymph-adenopathy
with glands above and below the inguinal ligament—**groove sign**.

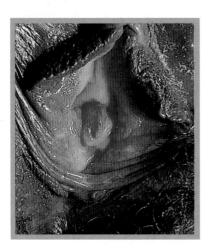

↑ 197 Lymphogranuloma venereum of vulva
Note considerable oedema.

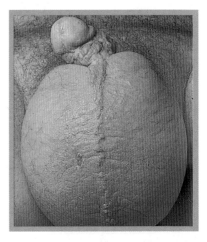

↑ 198 Lymphogranuloma venereum
Elephantiasis of scrotum.

COMMON INFLAMMATORY CONDITIONS

GONORRHEA

This universally common, highly contagious disease is a bacterial infection affecting columnar or transitional epithelium. It may, therefore, be found in the **urethra** or **rectum** in males; the **urethra**, **cervical canal** and **rectum** in females; the **pharynx** and **tonsils** in both sexes; the **conjunctival sac** (especially in the newborn) in both sexes; and in the **vagina** and **vulva** of prepubertal females. Local or metastatic spread occasionally occurs.

In most male cases, the disease is acute and complications resulting from local spread of the organism are rare. In females, the disease is frequently asymptomatic; in consequence, diagnosis and treatment are often delayed and local complications may be the cause of the patient's attendance.

In both sexes bacteraemia may occur and this results in metastatic involvement of remote tissues, e.g. skin lesions, septic arthritis or, very rarely, endocarditis or meningitis. In males, postgonococcal stricture of the urethra is now very rare. **It is important to remember that gonococcal infection often coexists with other sexually transmitted infections.**

The organism

The causative organism is the coccus *Neisseria gonorrhoeae*. It is usually identified in Gram-stained smears as an intracellular Gram-negative diplococcus. Positive distinction from other forms of Neisseria is made by the unique pattern of sugar fermentation reactions of organisms grown in culture. Differences in plasmids have also been observed, often associated with differences in antibiotic sensitivity. A small proportion of cases are due to other Neisseria species

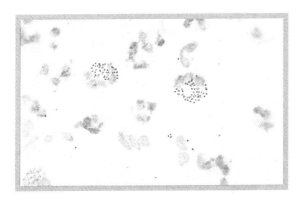

← **199 Gram-stained smear showing Gram-negative intra-cellular diplococci: *Neisseria gonor-rhoeae***

Incubation period

The incubation period of gonorrhoea is usually 4–7 days. Occasionally, the incubation period may be as little as 24 hours. Prolonged incubation of 1 month or more appears to becoming more common. In male patients, acute symptomatic disease makes determination of incubation easy in most cases, but in female patients and asymptomatic infections, this determination is impossible without epidemiological data.

Diagnosis

Gram-stained smears of material from affected sites are examined microscopically. In males, most cases can be diagnosed by this method but cultures should always be inoculated to find infections unrecognized on smears of urethral discharge. In female patients, smear diagnosis is less accurate and most infections can be demonstrated only by cultural methods. In addition, culture results can be used to show patterns of antibiotic sensitivity.

Fluorescent staining methods are also available, but are not currently used in clinical practice.

The gonococcal complement-fixation test (GCFT) is seldom helpful. Reports show that the test currently in use gives unacceptably high rates of false-negative and false-positive results. Considerable research is being undertaken to develop a more satisfactory serum test.

Uncomplicated gonorrhoea in males

Most infections cause acute symptomatic urethritis; asymptomatic urethritis is not uncommon (c. 5–10%) and appears to be increasing in frequency; signs may be easy or hard to detect. Gonococcal proctitis is found in anoreceptive homosexuals some of whom are found to have concurrent urethritis and/or pharyngitis.

Clinical course

Gonococcal urethritis; in most cases symptoms progress rapidly after onset. **Pain on urination** is frequent and may become extremely severe and cause retention of urine. **Urethral discharge** begins as scanty mucoid secretion which, in most cases, soon becomes copious and grossly purulent, and is sometimes bloodstained. Moderate **meatal oedema** and **balanoposthitis** are common, and painful **lymph gland enlargement** occurs in about 15% of cases. Slight to moderate oedema of the distal penile shaft and prepuce is frequently found and may be exacerbated by thrombosis of penile dorsal veins or lymphangitis. Rarely, gonococcal exudate may cause folliculitis or cellulitis on the thigh or abdomen. Anatomical anomalies such as paraurethral ducts or median raphe sinuses may sometimes be the site of gonococcal infection. The relative avascularity of these structures may make cure more difficult to achieve.

Gonococcal proctitis. Symptoms are often mild or absent: many patients found to have infection attend at the instigation of a partner who has developed gonococcal urethritis. Patients may complain of **anal dampness**, **pruritus** or **discomfort**, a mucoid or purulent **anal discharge** and, occasionally, **tenesmus**. White, yellow or bloodstained discharge may be noticed on the surface of the motions.

Proctoscopy may show normal mucosa or a variable degree of **proctitis**; inspection may show no discharge (even in cases later shown by smear or culture to be infected) or muco-pus may be seen. In severe cases, bloodstained purulent discharge is seen to be exuding from mucosal folds.

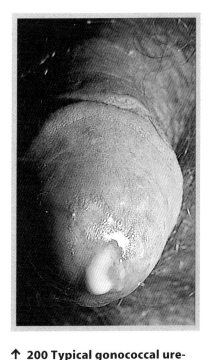

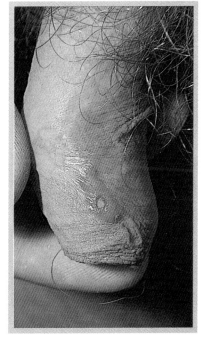

↑ **200 Typical gonococcal urethritis**
Note associated meatitis.

↑ **201 Gonorrhoea**
of median raphe sinus.

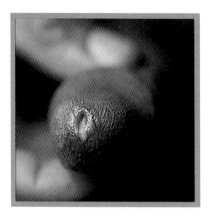

↑ **202 Gonocococcal meatitis.**

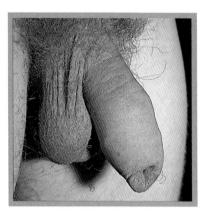

↑ **203 Gonococcal urethritis** with oedema of distal penile shaft.

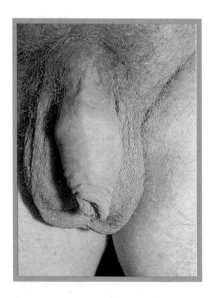

↑ **204 Gonococcal urethritis** with folliculitis of thigh (site of contact with meatus).

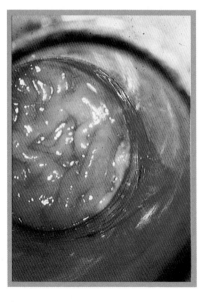

↑ **205 Gonococcal proctitis** Note oedema of mucosa.

Genital complications of gonorrhoea in males

Spread of gonococcal infection from the urethra to contiguous structures may occur in early infection, but such complications are now extremely rare (<0.5%) in developed countries. Involvement of local glandular structures (**Tyson's**, **Littre's**, **Cowper's** and **prostate**) or unilateral or bilateral **epididymitis** is occasionally seen. Rarely, gonococcal penile ulcers are found. Periurethral abscesses and fistulae are now almost unknown.

Urethral strictures developing long after gonococcal urethritis are still occasionally found but are now very uncommon in developed countries.

Local complications nearly always develop shortly after the appearance of the related urethritis; determination of the aetiology is usually easy. Occasionally, signs of urethritis may be slight and the infection difficult to diagnose. It has been observed that when the signs of epididymitis appear, the signs of urethritis often diminish. Rarely, this complication may be the only gonococcal lesion present.

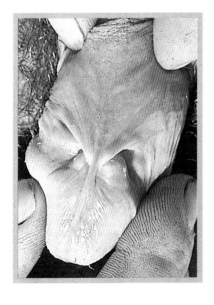

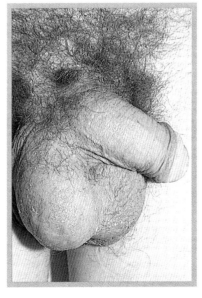

↑ **206 Gonococcal urethritis**
with tysonitis.

↑ **207 Gonococcal epididymitis.**

Uncomplicated gonorrhoea in females

Gonococcal infections in females may involve the **urethra, cervical canal or rectum**; any or all of the sites may be affected concurrently. Gonococcal proctitis in females may occur as a result of rectal intercourse or by autoinfection from infected vulval discharge. Proctitis may be resistant to treatment and may itself cause reinfection of the urethra or cervix.

Clinical course

Symptoms are **absent** or so **slight** that they are ignored by the patient in about 80% of cases, even in those patients who have recognizable signs of infection. Symptomatic patients most frequently complain of **urinary symptoms**—mild to severe pain on urination, dysuria and sometimes symptoms of cystitis. Slight or moderate increase in **vaginal secretion** may be noticed; the secretion may become discoloured, often yellow. Rectal symptoms occur as in male gonococcal proctitis. Rarely, there is painful enlargement of inguinal lymph nodes.

Signs of infection are very variable. Many patients with bacteriologically proved infection have a completely normal appearance when examined. Mucopurulent or purulent **urethral discharge** may be seen (even in the absence of urinary symptoms), and is often associated with oedema of the meatus. Ulceration of the meatal margin and involvement of Skene's glands is occasionally found. The cervix may appear normal with mucoid secretion or may show endocervicitis, varying from slight erythema around the os to extensive (2–3 cm diameter) granulating and purulent erosions. **Cervical discharge** is typically mucopurulent: in severe cases it may be profuse, frankly purulent and bloodstained. Signs of proctitis are as variable as in males with gonococcal proctitis.

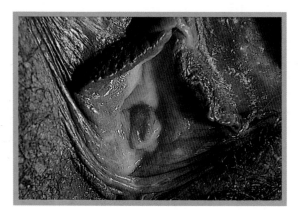

← **208 Gonococcal urethritis.**

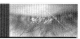
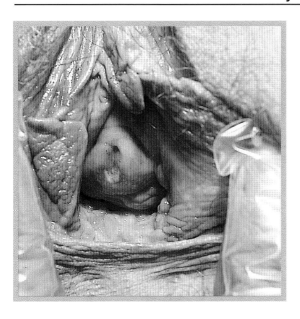

← 209
Gonorrhoea
Urethritis and
ulceration.

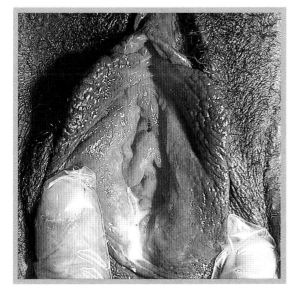

← 210
Gonorrhoea
Purulent 'vaginal'
discharge.

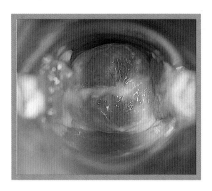

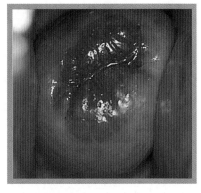

↑211 Gonorrhoea
Purulent cervical discharge and
exocervicitis

↑212 Gonorrhoea
Virtually normal cervix in which
gonorrhoea was found.

Genital complications of gonorrhoea in females

Complications of gonorrhoea are relatively much more common in females than in males. It has been estimated that the incidence is about 10%, and a considerable number of female patients are found to have gonorrhoea solely because of the development of symptoms or signs of complication. This high incidence is almost certainly because of the asymptomatic nature of most cases of early infection which may allow the infection to be present for a considerable time before manifestation, with consequent greater likelihood of local spread and complication.

Local spread may involve local glandular structures (**Skene's** and **Bartholin's**) or progress into or through the uterine cavity to cause **endometritis** or salpingitis (pelvic inflammatory disease—PID).

Bartholinitis may vary from slight painless enlargement of the gland, detected incidentally, to a surgical emergency with a grossly enlarged, exquisitely tender gland, with associated cutaneous oedema and erythema. Pus, in which gonococci can be found, may be expressed from the Bartholin's duct or may be obtained by aspiration or drainage of the gland. Following acute infection, Bartholin's cyst may occur.

The most serious complication of gonorrhoea is **salpingitis** (**pelvic inflammatory disease**) with possible sequelae of chronic pelvic infection, sterility and increased likelihood of ectopic pregnancy. Gonococcal salpingitis is very variable in severity, ranging from mild cases recognized during examination to severe cases presenting as acute abdominal emergencies. The diagnosis is clinical (sometimes made at laparotomy); the aetiology is determined by genital bacteriology which must include tests for coexistent infections such as chlamydia. Symptoms and signs include lower abdominal pain (often in one or both iliac fossae) and tenderness; prolonged and irregular menstruation or intermittent vaginal bleeding; deep dyspareunia; and, often, moderate pyrexia and malaise. Bimanual pelvic examination may reveal pain when the cervix is moved (the cervical excitation sign, the 'chandelier' sign see p. 37) or enlargement and tenderness of the Fallopian tubes. In severe cases, pelvic peritonitis may be present, and chronic pelvic infection may ensue.

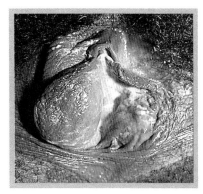

← 213 Gonorrhoea
Bartholin's abscess.

Disseminated gonococcal infection (metastatic gonorrhoea)

Neisseria gonorrhoeae, like any other pathogenic organism, can occasionally find its way into the bloodstream to produce bacteraemia and metastatic complications. Bacteraemia is considered more likely to occur in chronic cases or to follow instrumentation or manipulation of infected tissues. In most reported cases of disseminated infection, the genital focus has been present for 2–4 weeks at least, and may be asymptomatic. Reports in the past have probably incorrectly ascribed a gonococcal aetiology to patients with symptoms and findings of Reiter's syndrome, a complication of non-gonococcal urethritis.

Metastatic complications are rare and are mentioned only briefly: **septic arthritis**, **tenosynovitis**, **endocarditis**, **meningitis**, **skin lesions**. Skin lesions are the commonest complication, usually seen on the extremities but occasionally on the trunk. The lesions are transient; they begin as sparse erythematous papules and progress to vesicles or pustules which heal without scarring after a few days. The skin lesions are usually only slightly painful.

127

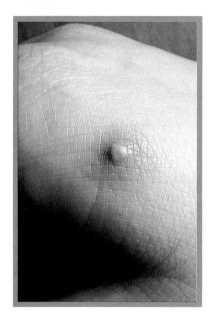 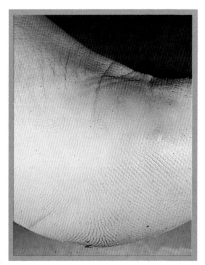

↑ 214, 215 Disseminated gonococcal infection
214 Vesicopustule on dorsum of hand. **215** Less florid lesion on the foot.

Other sites of gonococcal infection— pharynx and tonsils, conjunctival sac

Recent reports show an increasing frequency of gonorrhoea affecting the pharynx and tonsils, apparently linked with an increase in orogenital contact (cunnilingus, fellatio). The infection may very occasionally be communicated by oral contact (kissing) alone. Genitourinary gonorrhoea can usually be found as well; in some cases the disease is confined to the oral cavity. The infection is often asymptomatic and discovered only by examination. In some patients, symptoms of pharyngitis or tonsillitis occur: examination may show diffuse pharyngitis, follicular tonsillitis or, occasionally, ulceration of the throat or tonsil. Moderate cervical lymph gland enlargement is common. The diagnosis must be established by careful bacteriological examination, including sugar fermentation reactions, or by fluorescent methods, as other organisms frequently found in the oral cavity or pharynx may resemble gonococci on smears.

Gonorrhoea is one of the causes of **ophthalmia neonatorum**: it is now rare in developed countries. Signs of the infection usually appear 2–5 days after delivery, affecting one or both eyes. The infant becomes photophobic and mucoid discharge appears at the lid margins, rapidly becoming profuse, sometimes bloodstained. The eyelids become swollen and erythematous; subcutaneous haemorrhages may appear. The tarsal conjunctiva shows oedema and intense injection; the bulbar conjunctiva shows injection; subconjunctival haemorrhages are common. In advanced cases corneal ulceration, corneal perforation and panophthalmitis may occur. The infection is acquired during delivery from unrecognized maternal gonococcal endocervicitis; it is essential for the mother and her partner(s) to be examined. The course of conjunctivitis in adults is essentially the same as in infants. The disease is usually acquired by accidental inoculation (often autoinoculation) of infectious material from genitourinary gonorrhoea.

Vulvovaginitis
Before puberty, the vulval and vaginal epithelium is susceptible to gonococcal infection. After puberty, the hormonal changes causing cornification of the epithelium diminish the susceptibility. Contact with *N. gonorrhoeae* by young females may cause vulvovaginitis. In infants, the infection may be acquired during delivery, but carryover of maternal oestrogens usually causes the epithelium to be temporarily resistant. In older girls, infection may be acquired by sexual contact (sometimes not admitted or not realized); or accidentally from fomites (e.g. rectal thermometers); from non-sexual contact with infected adults; the possibility of child abuse should never be overlooked. The infection may present with vulval soreness, painful urination, or discharge on underclothing. Examination shows purulent vaginal discharge and vulvitis, and often considerable oedema. Careful bacteriological tests are essential to distinguish gonococcal infection from other causes of vulvovaginitis. When gonococcal vulvovaginitis is found, it is important to trace the source, who may be asymptomatic and unaware of the disease.

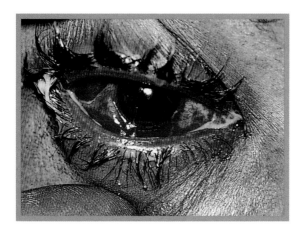

← **216 Gonococcal ophthalmia**
Subconjunctival haemorrhages.

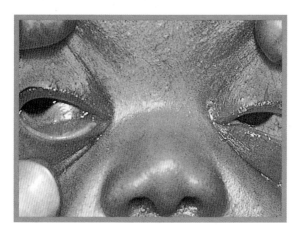

← **217 Gonococcal ophthalmia**
Infant, showing marked oedema of lids.

NON-GONOCOCCAL GENITAL INFECTION

Non-gonococcal genital infection is common and in many parts of the developed world, non-gonococcal urethritis (NGU) is much more frequent than gonorrhoea. Most cases of non-gonococcal genital infection are mild but complications include **salpingitis (pelvic inflammatory disease (PID))** in women, **epididymitis** in men and **sexually acquired reactive arthritis (SARA)** in both sexes; the more fulminant manifestations of the latter being termed **Reiter's syndrome**.

It is now known that men, as well as women, are often asymptomatic, sometimes for long periods, and it is thus important to investigate and treat all partners to prevent recurrence of infection. Rectal and oral carriage of organisms in homosexual men may also be asymptomatic.

Urethritis in male patients (and corresponding conditions in female patients) can be simply divided into two categories: **gonococcal** and **non-gonococcal**. The former has already been dealt with in the preceding section. **Non-gonococcal urethritis (NGU)** can be further subdivided into groups with known aetiology and unknown aetiology. Research suggests a probable or possible cause for about 70% of cases of NGU (see **220**), most commonly *C. trachomatis*. In the remaining 30% of cases, no cause can be identified. In clinical practice—without comprehensive microbiology—over half the time no cause can be found when the condition has loosely been termed **non-specific urethritis (NSU)**, with the female equivalent known as **non-specific cervicitis (NSC)**; the term 'non-specific genital infection' (**NSGI**) is used for both sexes. **Non-specific proctitis** also occurs. The epidemiology of non-specific genital infections is often very suggestive of sexual transmission and although various organisms (e.g. mycoplasmas, including ureaplasmas) have been suggested as aetiological agents, it has been difficult to establish definite links.

Two further conditions have also to be considered in this section: **acute haemorrhagic cystitis** and **chronic prostatitis**.

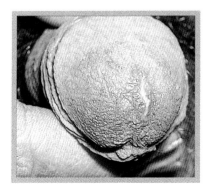

← 218 Non-gonococcal urethritis
Typical mucopurulent discharge.

Microbial

Chlamydia trachomatis	30%–50%
Ureaplasma urealyticum	?10%–30%
Neither of the above	20%–40%
Mycoplasma genitalium	?5%–10%
Bacteria: aerobes/anaerobes	none substantiated
Viruses: Herpes simplex	<1%
Yeasts	<1%
Parasites: *Trichomonas vaginalis*	<3%
Secondary to upper urinary tract infection	
Secondary to intraurethral lesions	
e.g. chancre, warts	

Non-microbial

Secondary to physical or chemical trauma

↑ **219 Aetiology of non-gonococcal urethritis.**

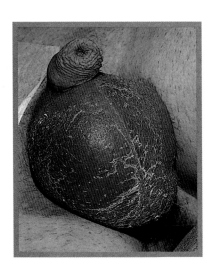

← **220 Non-gonococcal epididymitis**
with inflammatory hydrocele and erythema of scrotum.

Clinical course

In **males**, the incubation period of urethritis is usually 2–4 weeks. Some infections present within a few days of contact and in mild cases the symptoms may not be noticed for several months, especially if intermittent.

Symptoms are usually mild but are occasionally severe. Some cases are completely asymptomatic and are detected only on routine examination; occasionally the development of a complication is the first sign of infection. **Urinary symptoms** vary from mild meatal irritation to severe dysuria, with or without urgency and frequency of urination. **Urethral discharge** is usually noticed by the patient, but in mild cases may be detected only after the urine has been retained overnight. The discharge is usually mucoid or mucopurulent, but occasionally may simulate typical gonococcal urethritis. Associated **balanoposthitis** and local **lymphadenopathy** are uncommon. Rarely, local complications, such as **epididymitis**, may occur; urethral stricture very occasionally develops later. Following resolution of urethritis, prostatic fluid often shows excessive numbers of leucocytes, but it is uncertain whether this finding is primary or secondary.

In anoreceptive homosexual patients, **non-gonococcal proctitis** may be found. This is usually asymptomatic but may cause rectal discharge or tenesmus.

In **females**, complete absence of symptoms and recognizable abnormal findings on examination is usual. Occasionally, the development of a complication such as **Bartholinitis** or **pelvic inflammatory disease (PID)** (see below) indicates the presence of NSGI.

Occasionally, patients may present with upper abdominal pain caused by **perihepatitis (Fitz–Hugh–Curtis syndrome)**.

Aetiology of salpingitis		
C. trachomatis		40–60%
N. gonorrhoeae		5–15%
Anaerobes		5–10%
Mycoplasma:	M. hominis	5–10%
	M. genitalium	5–10%
Other		20%

← **221** Aetiology of salpingitis.

Diagnosis

Gram-stained urethral smears taken from males with NGU show leucocytes and epithelial cells, and may be either abacterial or contain normal urethral commensal organisms; the 'two glass' test shows anterior urethral involvement. Results from cultures and other laboratory investigations are usually only available 4–7 days after receipt of the specimens; these results may reveal a cause (e.g. *C. trachomatis*) but frequently show no recognized pathogens (i.e. NSGI). In female patients, leucocytes are often seen in urethral and cervical smears, but diagnostic criteria have not been established to indicate whether these findings have significance.

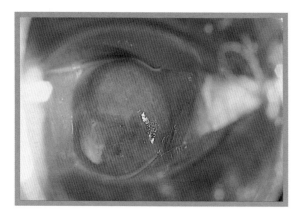

← 222 Non-gonococcal cervicitis.

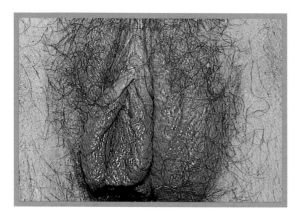

← 224 Non-specific infection
Bartholinitis.

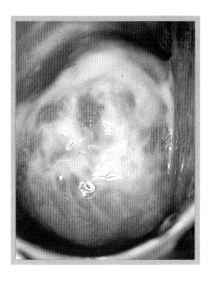

↑ 223 Non-gonococcal cervicitis.

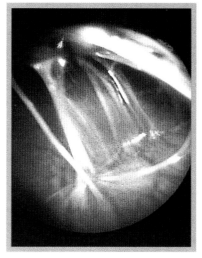

↑ 225 Perihepatitis
(Fitz–Hugh–Curtis syndrome)
Inactive disease showing 'violin
string' adhesions between liver
capsule and diaphragm.

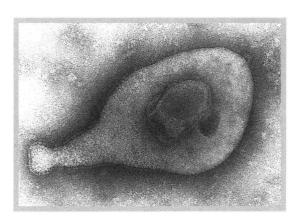

← 226
Mycoplasmum
genitalium.

Chlamydial infection

Chlamydiae were first identified in conjunctival scrapings in 1907 by Halberstabter and Prowazek; research soon showed similar intracellular organisms could be found in the pharynx, urethra, cervix and rectum. At first, little clinical research was possible because culture and other diagnostic methods were not available. Successful culture techniques were developed in the 1960s. Initially these were used only in research laboratories but, since the 1980s, diagnostic techniques (culture and more recently non-cultural antigen detection techniques) have become widely available. From using sensitive and specific tests, it is now realized that about 50% of cases formerly diagnosed as NSGI are caused by *C. trachomatis* and that chlamydial infections are the commonest sexually transmitted disease in developed countries.

Cause

C. trachomatis is an obligate intracellular microorganism. The trachoma biovar consists of serovars A, B and C, which are associated with trachoma, while serovars D to K are associated with urogenital disease, inclusion conjunctivitis (adult chlamydial ophthalmia and ophthalmia neonatorum) and neonatal pneumonia. The LGV biovar, serovars 1, 2 and 3, cause **lymphogranuloma venereum**. The LGV biovar can also cause proctitis but there is no good evidence that non-LGV (trachoma) serovars commonly cause rectal inflammation.

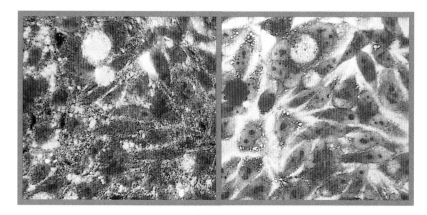

↑ 227 Cell culture of *C. trachomatis*
Two identical sections. Right, H&E stain; left, chlamydial inclusions fluoresce under dark-ground illumination.

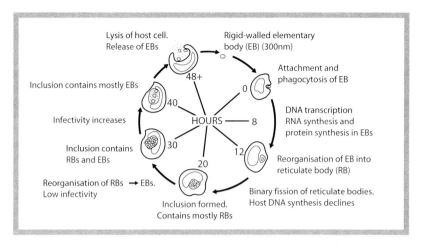

Lysis of host cell.
Release of EBs

Rigid-walled elementary
body (EB) (300nm)

Attachment and
phagocytosis of EB

Inclusion contains mostly EBs

DNA transcription
RNA synthesis and
protein synthesis in EBs

Infectivity increases

HOURS

Reorganisation of EB into
reticulate body (RB)

Inclusion contains
RBs and EBs

Binary fission of reticulate bodies.
Host DNA synthesis declines

Reorganisation of RBs → EBs.
Low infectivity

Inclusion formed.
Contains mostly RBs

48+ 0 8 12 20 30 40

↑ **228 Life cycle of *Chlamydia trachomatis*.**

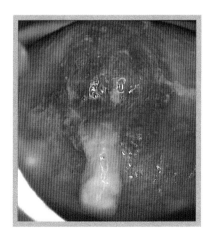

↑ **229 Chlamydial cervicitis.**

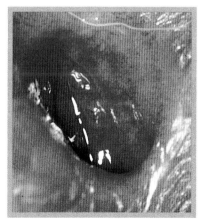

↑ **230 Chlamydia**
Urethral meatus showing meatitis,
papillary congestion and follicular
lesions.

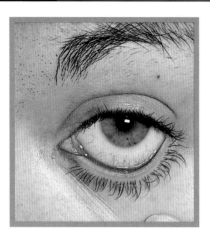

← 231 Mild chlamydial conjunctivitis.

Incubation period

In males with chlamydial urethritis, the incubation period ranges from 3–30 days; commonly 10–21 days. In females, the usually asymptomatic pattern of uncomplicated infection makes the incubation period difficult to determine: there is no reason to suppose that if differs from the pattern seen in males.

Diagnosis

There has been a rapid expansion in the number of techniques available for the detection of chlamydial organisms. Culture, in the best hands, is a most satisfactory technique, but requires special facilities, is time-consuming and therefore is expensive. Over recent years, ELISA techniques have been popular as transport is easier and specimens may be batched, but unfortunately many of these techniques have been somewhat non-specific and lacking in sensitivity. More recently, polymerase chain reaction and a variant, ligase chain reaction, have shown excellent sensitivity and specificity.

For rapid diagnosis of one-off specimens, a direct immunofluorescence test to detect elementary bodies in smears is useful but requires an expert observer.

Serological tests to detect antibodies (including the sensitive micro-immunofluorescence) add little in routine clinical practice. The LGV/psittacosis complement fixation test is supportive of the diagnosis in patients who clinically have lymphogranuloma venereum (see page 116).

Acute haemorrhagic cystitis

The condition present as non-specific urethritis associated with haematuria (often gross) and severe symptoms of cystitis. The cause is unknown but the clinical pattern suggests that the condition is a separate entity.

Chronic prostatitis

The definition, diagnosis and effects of this condition are all vague as the symptomatology may occur in patients with normal physical findings, and abnormalities in the prostatic fluid may be found in apparently normal individuals. Findings designated as chronic prostatitis are often found in patients with **Reiter's syndrome**, **anterior uveitis** and **ankylosing spondylitis** but the relationship of the prostatic symptoms to the other findings is not understood. Chronic prostatitis may be a sequel to urethritis of any aetiology and it seems probable some cases of apparently NSU are in fact exacerbations of chronic prostatitis.

The diagnosis is usually based on examination of the prostatovesicular secretions expressed by prostatic massage (see p. 53). Prostatic fluid is collected on a slide (or series of slides) and examined microscopically. Abnormal prostatic fluid shows excessive numbers of leucocytes (>5 per high-power field) which are often clumped. Very rarely, organisms such as *Trichomonas vaginalis* and bacteria may be identified. Unfortunately, similar findings are not uncommon in apparently normal individuals and it is usually difficult to correlate clinical symptoms and findings with results of prostatic fluid examination. Ultrasound imaging, particularly with a rectal probe, may help in clarifying the diagnosis: prostatic biopsy may also be used.

The symptoms associated with chronic prostatitis include meatal discomfort, pain passing from the perineum to meatus, and aching in the testes and perineum, all often aggravated by ejaculation. Mucoid urethral discharge may occur, especially after defaecation. Urinary symptoms include mild obstruction and urethral itching during micturition. Discoloration of the ejaculate (rusty or red colours) from haematospermia is common and may be the presenting symptom. Other patients notice yellow mucoid lumps in the ejaculate. Paradoxically, many patients with these symptoms have apparently normal prostatic findings on examination.

The findings on examination include slight enlargement of the prostate (and often of the seminal vesicles also) traditionally with a 'boggy' or 'nodular' feel, but such findings may occur in asymptomatic men or with normal microscopical examination of the expressed prostatic fluid in cases with symptomatology suggestive of chronic prostatitis.

Sexually acquired reactive arthritis (SARA) and Reiter's syndrome (Feissinger–Leroy syndrome)
Reactive arthritis may be secondary to an SARA infection or to a gastrointestinal infection, as in the original description by Reiter of patients with dysentery. Classically, Reiter's syndrome is a triad of **non-gonococcal genital infection**, **arthritis** and **conjunctivitis** with frequent involvement of the skin and mucous membranes. However, the classical syndrome is comparatively rare and it is probable that many cases with incomplete forms of the syndrome go unrecognized. These would include patients with mild genital infection and ensethopathy (inflammation around the tendon insertion). Reiter's syndrome has a marked tendency to relapse after the initial attack has cleared up. Relapses may feature one or more of the manifestations and are not necessarily related to further episodes of genital inflammation.

Reactive arthritis develops in 1–2% of patients with non-gonococcal genital infections, with chlamydiae being the precipitating cause in over half the cases. However, the fullblown Reiter's syndrome is seen in less than 1% of NSGI and both are recognized less often in females. This may be because the genital infection is usually overt in males and covert in females, who may present with non-genital features of the syndrome in other clinical settings. The pathogenesis has still not been fully elucidated, but the condition is more common in patients who are HLA-B27 positive.

Diagnosis
The diagnosis of Reiter's syndrome is clinical and radiological. There is, at present, no laboratory investigation which is diagnostic, but investigations can positively exclude other conditions which may be confused with Reiter's syndrome.

Clinical course
In most cases, the first indications of Reiter's syndrome are the appearance of conjunctivitis and/or arthritis within 1–2 weeks after the onset of genital infection. Unfortunately, the preceding genital infection has no particular features which enable Reiter's syndrome to be identified in advance, and the severity of the genital infection bears no relationship to the severity of subsequent Reiter's syndrome. The clinical course is very variable; although most cases are mild, severe systemic disorder is occasionally seen. The disease has protean manifestations which are outlined below. In addition to localized symptoms and signs, systemic abnormalities are often found. In many patients, there is moderate fever and the erythrocyte sedimentation rate (ESR) is raised, sometimes to 100 mm or more per hour in episodes of disease activity.

Genital infection

The non-gonococcal genital infection found may present as **urethritis, cervicitis, cystitis** or **prostatitis**. Sometimes the infection is asymptomatic and detected only on careful examination. Occasionally extragenital manifestations of Reiter's syndrome may precede signs of the genital infection.

Visceral lesions

Thrombophlebitis, peripheral neuritis, myocarditis, aortic incompetence and secondary amyloidosis have occasionally been described in patients with Reiter's syndrome: all are rare. Very rarely, other types of systemic involvement have been reported.

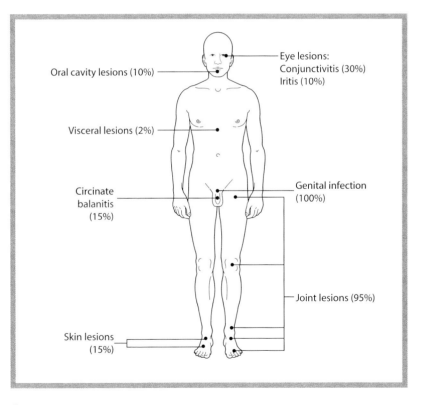

↑ 232 The manifestations of Reiter's syndrome.

Joint lesions

About 95% of patients with Reiter's syndrome develop lesions in the joints or adjacent tissues. Usually, objective changes of arthritis are found but in some patients **arthralgia** is the only abnormal skeletal manifestation. **Arthritis** usually appears in the course of the first episode but may become evident only in a later relapse. With repeated relapses, considerable permanent change may occur, often involving the metatarsophalangeal joints or causing spur formation beneath or behind the os calcis. Occasionally, spinal changes, difficult to differentiate from ankylosing spondylitis, may develop. The arthritis is usually polyarticular, often more or less symmetrical and particularly likely to affect the peripheral joints of the lower limbs; the sacroiliac, knee, ankle and foot joints are most commonly involved. Monoarticular arthritis may occur and is seen most often in the knee. The arthritis is non-suppurative and may be either acute or subacute. When it is acute, the process may spread to involve adjacent soft tissues, seen most often in the plantar fascia or Achilles tendon. In most attacks, the arthritis clears up after 4–6 weeks. Relapses are usually shorter in duration and milder, but with successive attacks increasing deformity is likely to develop.

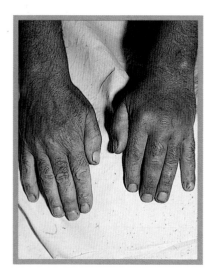

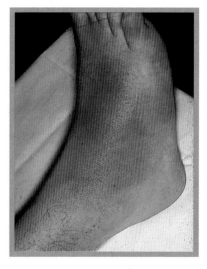

↑ **233 Reiter's syndrome**
Arthritis of left hand, principally affecting metacarpophalangeal joints.

↑ **234 Reiter's syndrome**
Arthritis of foot. Note involvement of mid-foot, ankle and metatarsals.

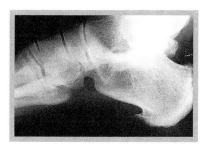

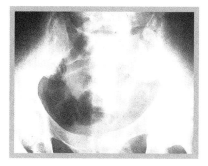

↑ **235 Reiter's syndrome**
Radiograph of foot. Note inferior calcaneal spur and deformity of metatarsophalangeal joints. Note also posterior calcaneal erosions.

↑ **236 Reiter's syndrome**
Radiograph of sacroiliac joints. Note sclerosis on left side.

Eye lesions

Conjunctivitis occurs in about 30% of patients with Reiter's syndrome and is often the first indication of the condition. It is usually mild and transient but may occasionally be severe and associated with chemosis. One or both eyes may be involved. The tarsal conjunctiva tends to be more severely affected, especially at the lateral angles. Relapses are common, and conjunctivitis is frequently the only lesion in a relapse.

Iritis occurs in about 10% of patients. It may initially be found late in the first attacks of Reiter's syndrome or may only appear weeks or months after initial symptoms; relapses are very common. Synechiae formed in repeated attacks can cause secondary glaucoma which may endanger vision; iridectomy is sometimes necessary to preserve sight.

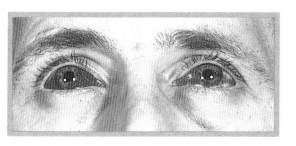

← **237 Reiter's syndrome**
Severe bilateral conjunctivitis with chemosis. Such severity is unusual.

Skin lesions

Keratoderma blennorrhagica occurs in about 15% of patients, often in the more severe cases with many signs, but is occasionally seen alone. The rash is found most characteristically on the soles of the feet. It may be found elsewhere on the skin or scalp, and in particularly severe cases the nails and nail-beds are likely to be involved. Typical lesions occur on the penis in circumcised males. The lesions begin as discrete small subcutaneous papules which become vesicular and covered with a heaped-up adherent crust. Spreading lesions become confluent and may involve extensive areas. Subungual lesions may cause lifting or loss of the nail.

Circinate balanitis is seen on the glans penis and prepuce in uncircumcised males. Small, discrete, round or oval red macules or shallow erosions appear which often spread centrifugally and become confluent. The topography of the confluent lesions is circinate and the margin is often slightly elevated and grey in colour. About 15% of patients with Reiter's syndrome have this lesion.

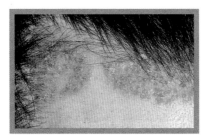

← **238 Keratoderma blennorrhagica**
of forehead and scalp.

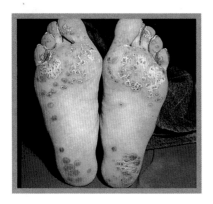

← **239 Keratoderma blennorrhagica**
of feet.

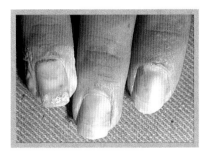

← 240
Keratoderma
Lesions on hand and foot.

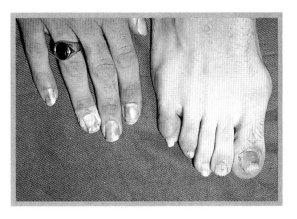

↑ **241 Keratoderma**
Close-up of finger lesions seen in **240.**

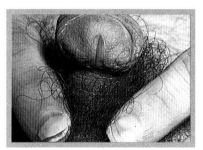

↑ **242 Keratoderma**
of penis and fingers.

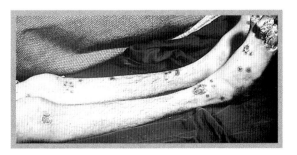

← 243
Keratoderma
of legs. Note also joint swelling from arthritis.

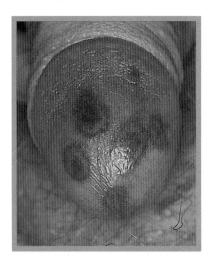

↑ **244 Reiter's syndrome**
Circinate balanitis.

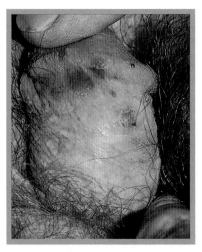

↑ **245 Keratoderma**
of penis.

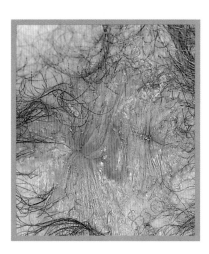

↑ **246 Reiter's syndrome**
Perianal lesions.

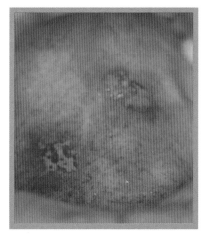

↑ **247 Reiter's syndrome**
Lesions on palate.

Oral lesions

Small painless vesicular or erosive lesions are found in the oral cavity in about 10% of patients with Reiter's syndrome. Lesions are commonly seen on the tongue (dorsum and edge) or palate, but may also occur elsewhere in the oral cavity. The surface of the lesion may be erythematous or covered with grey exudate. This exudate is often thicker at the margin of the lesion.

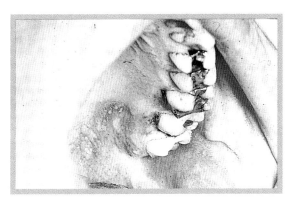

← **248 Reiter's syndrome**
Lesions on buccal mucosa.

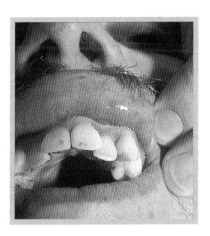

↑ **249 Reiter's syndrome**
Lesions on lip.

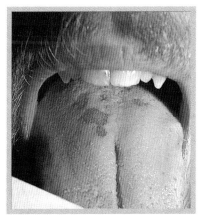

↑ **250 Reiter's syndrome**
Lesions on tongue.

CANDIDIASIS (THRUSH)

Candida albicans (*Monilia*) infection is the most common fungal infection encountered in genitourinary practice. Genital dermatomycosis may also be caused by other *Candida* species (which are not discussed separately) or to the other fungal infections described on p. 202). Thrush may be transmitted or exacerbated by sexual contact, but most infections (particularly in women) result from autoinoculation from the rectum. Symptoms may be caused by hypersensitivity or infection. If caused by hypersensitivity alone, microbiological investigations are negative. The fungus is frequently found as an asymptomatic saprophyte in the mouth, colon, rectum and genital region. Symptomatic infections are much less common and may be caused by the intervention of another factor. These other factors include pregnancy, glycosuria, antibiotic or immunosuppressive therapy, and oral contraceptives: physical factors such as obesity, tight clothing and hyperhydrosis may be significant. In clinical practice, the condition may present with symptoms in one partner only, but it is essential to examine the asymptomatic partner to reduce the chance of reinfection. Severe problems with Candida may occur in immunodeficient patients, e.g. people with HIV infection. In such patients, the oral cavity is often seriously affected; infection may extend into the oesophagus and occasionally to other parts of the alimentary canal (see p. 308).

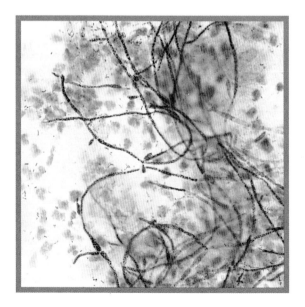

← 251 Hyphae of *Candida albicans* in vaginal smear. Gram stain.

The organism

Candida albicans may be found in either mycelial (hyphae) and/or spore forms. Mixed forms are common; the spores are often seen to be budding. In Gram-stained smears taken from appropriate sites, *C. albicans* is nearly always Gram-positive. The fungus may also be identified on culture, which is more sensitive.

Diagnosis

The diagnosis is made by demonstration of the causative organism, *C. albicans*, either on smear or on culture. The organism may also be recognized on cervical cytological smears. The material for examination may be taken from any of the sites liable to be affected. It should be remembered that symptoms suggestive of candidiasis may be caused by contact dermatitis; these patients will be microbiologically negative. It is essential to **examine for glycosuria** as candidiasis is a not infrequent presentation of diabetes.

Clinical course

Asymptomatic or symptomatic infections may be found; both are more frequent in women. The incubation period is impossible to determine as asymptomatic carriage is so common. Sometimes symptoms may appear within minutes of sexual contact (as a result of hypersensitivity) or may be delayed for several days while infection develops.

Candidiasis in women

The pattern is very variable and symptoms and findings are often discordant: all symptoms are likely to be exacerbated by/around menstruation. **Irritation** (**pruritus**) almost always occurs in symptomatic cases which usually affects the **labia** and **vulva**. It may also affect the perineum, natal cleft and groins. Lumpy **vaginal discharge**, scanty or copious, is another very common symptom. **Swelling** of the labia and superficial dyspareunia are less frequent symptoms; occasionally a **rash** of the labia, pubis or groins is noted. Some women notice a change in **genital odour,** complaining of a **'sour'** smell.

Findings on examination are equally variable. The labia are often mildly or moderately **oedematous** (especially in chronic cases) and may be **erythematous**. **Intertrigo** often extends to the perianal region and occasionally to the groins. Follicular lesions may be seen, especially at the edges of involved areas. **Vulvitis** may be mild or severe; there is frequently associated **vaginitis** but either may be seen alone. Plaques of typical yellowish cheesy exudate may be seen on the vulva, vagina and cervix. Vaginal discharge may be typical or may be thin and grey. Shallow erosions, usually caused by scratching, may be found on the labia and perineum.

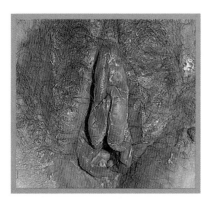

↑ **252 Candidiasis**
Vulvitis. Note the oedema (cf. with trichomoniasis, **280**).

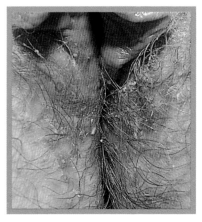

↑ **253 Candidiasis**
Note follicular lesions.

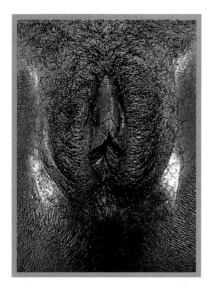

← **254 Candidiasis**
Chronic infection showing oedema, lichenification and extensive hyperpigmentation of upper thighs.

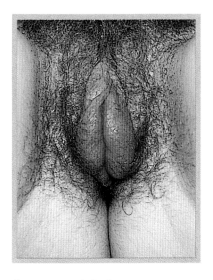

↑ 255 Candidiasis
Note oedema.

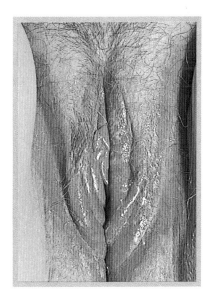

↑ 256 Candidiasis
Vulvitis with typical 'cheesy' plaques.

← 257 Candidiasis
Vulvitis and crural intertrigo.

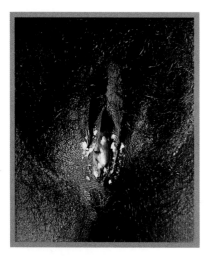

← 258 Candidiasis
Note Bartholinitis (antibiotic-treated) and 'cheesy' plaques of discharge.

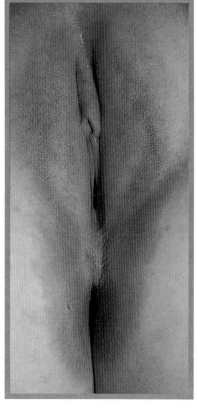

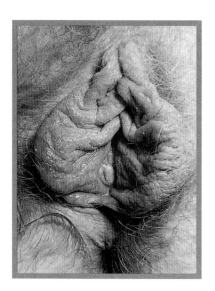

↑ 259 Candidiasis
Vulvitis: note the oedema and the grey mucoid discharge.

↑ 260 Candidiasis
In child.

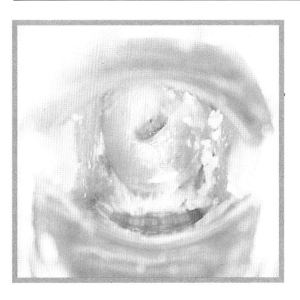

← 261
Candidiasis
Vaginitis with typical plaques of exudate on the cervix and vaginal wall.

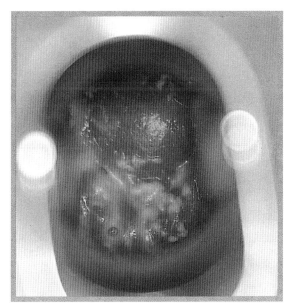

← 262
Candidiasis
Vaginitis, with exocervicitis and plaques of typical exudate on vaginal wall.

Candidiasis in men

The most common complaint is **pruritus (itching)** of the glans and prepuce, often associated with a **rash** and **swelling** of the affected parts. Occasionally, the pruritic rash may affect the pubis, scrotum or groins and, in homosexual patients, the perianal region. Symptoms of urethritis with marked meatal and distal urethral irritation occasionally occur; other symptoms are rare. Uncircumcised men are more likely to be affected.

Examination shows follicular or diffuse erythema of the glans and prepuce, frequently most marked in the coronal sulcus. Lesions in uncircumcised patients are moist, but in circumcised patients they are often dry and show a typical fungal centrifugal pattern. Scaling of the skin or mucous membrane and mucopurulent exudate are often seen; typical plaques are less common. Diffuse erythema of the scrotum and groin, often with marginal folliculitis, is occasionally seen. Urethritis may be found and is almost always mild. Candidiasis in association with HIV infection is discussed elsewhere (see p. 308).

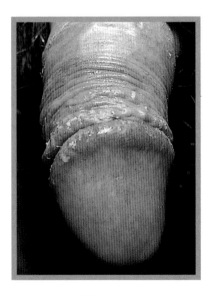

↑ **263 Candidiasis**
Balanoposthitis. A dry lesion showing 'glazed' oedematous mucosa and superficial fissuring.

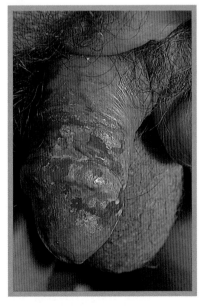

↑ **264 Candidiasis**
Severe infection.

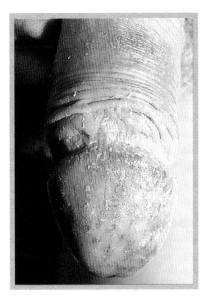

← 265 Candidiasis
Balanoposthitis. Dry lesion showing desquamation and white exudate.

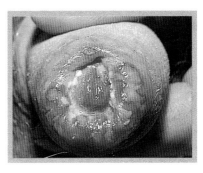

↑ 266 Candidiasis
Associated with herpes and phimosis (cf. secondary syphilis, **166**).

← 267 Candidiasis
Severe infection causing phimosis.

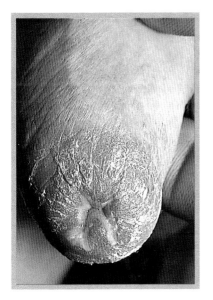

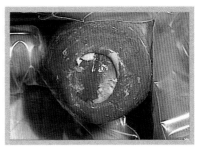

↑ 268 Candidiasis
Balanoposthitis. A diabetic patient presented with this lesion. His random blood sugar was 12.4 mmol/l. Note the typical plaques.

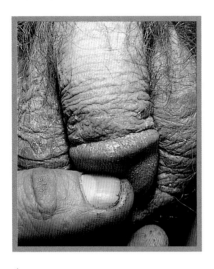

↑ **269 Candidiasis**
Penis and scrotum.

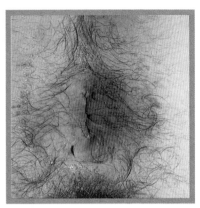

↑ **270 Candidiasis**
Perianal infection in anoreceptive homosexual. Note the peripheral satellite lesions. This patient's penetrative partner had candidal balanoposthitis.

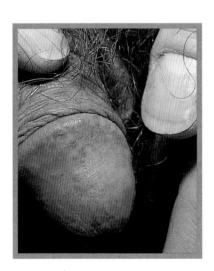

↑ **271 Candidiasis**
Glans penis and nails.

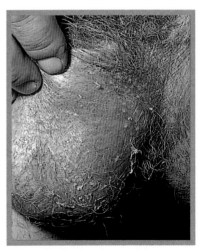

↑ **272 Candidiasis**
Intertrigo of scrotum and groin.

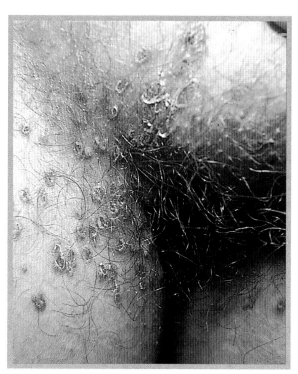

← 273
Candidiasis
Satellite pustules at periphery of groin lesion.

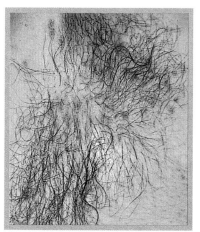

← 274 Candidiasis
Axilla.

TRICHOMONIASIS

Trichomonas vaginalis is a protozoal parasite which may be found in the vagina or urethra in women and the urethra or preputial sac in men; it is occasionally found in other genitourinary locations. The infestation may be asymptomatic or may cause acute or subacute inflammatory changes. It is probable that the parasite is usually transmitted sexually but accidental infection can occur. It seems likely that in some cases diagnosed in young female adolescents latent infestation has been present since birth. In women the duration of infestation is usually prolonged in the absence of treatment; in men infestation is often transient. In clinical practice, this is reflected by the condition being found 20 times more frequently in women. Trichomoniasis is frequently associated with other genitourinary disorders and it is essential to undertake examination to exclude such conditions.

The organism

Trichomonas vaginalis is a rounded or oval unicellular organism 15–30 μm in length; giant forms have occasionally been found. Four motile flagella project at the anterior end and an undulating membrane extends along the side of the body towards the projecting axostyle. The organism reproduces by fission.

Diagnosis

The parasite is most easily recognized in fresh microscopical specimens. Secretions from the posterior vaginal fornix and/or the urethra in women or from the urethra in men are mixed with a drop of saline on a slide. The specimen is covered with a cover slip or examined by a hanging drop technique. Microscopy, using dark-ground or reduced transmitted illumination, clearly shows the actively beating flagella and the undulating membrane. In affected women, the parasite is usually abundant; in affected men it may be sparse, and the diagnostic accuracy may be improved by instilling a few drops of saline into the terminal urethra, massaging the area and collecting the expressed fluid for examination.

Staining techniques are unsuitable for routine clinic use, but many unsuspected cases are found when the parasite is recognized in cervical exfoliative cytological smears. Cultures, using suitable media, inoculated with material taken from the usual sites of infestation, add considerably to the number of cases found by microscopy.

Clinical course

In acute and subacute cases, the incubation period appears to average 1–2 weeks. In asymptomatic cases, this is impossible to determine, and it is usually impossible to distinguish between latent infestation becoming active and newly acquired infection. Some infestations become evident when another type of infection is superimposed or after trauma to asymptomatic, infested sites. Pregnancy appears to predispose towards infection.

Trichomoniasis in women

Symptoms and findings are extremely variable and not necessarily correlated. Severe symptoms may be associated with almost normal findings and vice versa, with the fastidiousness of the individual patient being an important factor. The gradually increasing symptoms in prolonged infections may be regarded by the patients as 'normal,' even when grossly abnormal signs are found on examination. Common symptoms include: increased **vaginal discharge** (sometimes noticed only immediately before or after menstruation); **vulval soreness** and **superficial dyspareunia**; **offensive odour**; **vulval** and/or **perivulval pruritis**; **vulval** or **labial swelling**; and, occasionally, symptoms of urethritis or cystitis, mild pelvic discomfort and aching in the groins.

Examination findings are equally variable. **Vulvitis**, **vulval erosions**, **labial oedema**, **urethritis** and **vaginitis** are frequently found and **perivulvitis** is common; groin intertrigo is occasionally seen. In severe cases, the vaginal walls and cervix show the classical **'strawberry'** appearance with punctate bleeding erosions; in less acute infections, there is diffuse erythema of the exocervix. Vaginal discharge is most typically thin, frothy and purulent, but all types of vaginal discharge (mucoid, mucopurulent or grossly purulent and bloodstained) may be observed; the discharge is usually alkaline and between pH7 and pH9. Some urethral discharge is often present, and Bartholin's and Skene's glands are occasionally involved.

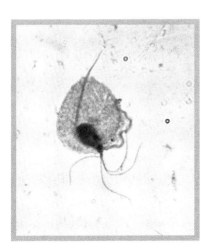

← 275 *Trichomonas vaginalis*
Note the pyriform shape, the four flagella, the lateral undulating membrane, the axostyle and the single nucleus.

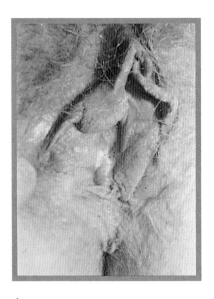

↑ **276 Trichomoniasis**
Typical vulvitis. Note the classical
frothy purulent discharge.

↑ **277 Trichomoniasis**
Dark-ground preparation showing
T. vaginalis and epithelial cells.

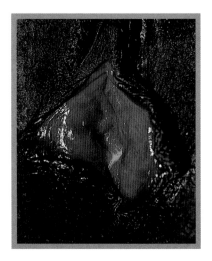

← **278 Trichomoniasis**
Acute vulvitis.

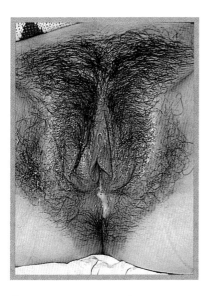

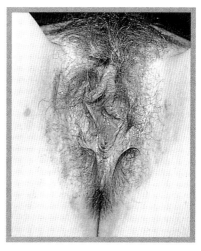

↑ 280 Trichomoniasis
Perivulvitis with urticarial lesions on the thigh and vulval oedema. Compare with **252** (candidal perivulvitis).

↑ 279 Trichomoniasis
Vulvitis, severe perivulvitis and perianal intertrigo.

← 281 Trichomoniasis
chronic.

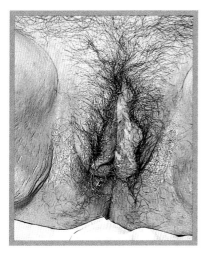

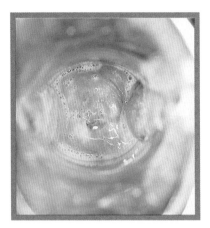

← 282 Trichomoniasis
Vaginitis and exocervicitis with classical frothy discharge.

Trichomoniasis in men
The infestation may be asymptomatic and diagnosed only when careful examination is made. Symptomatic cases usually present as **non-gonococcal urethritis**, clinically indistinguishable from NGU from other causes. Rarely, *T. vaginalis* may cause **balanoposthitis, prostatitis** or **epididymitis**. Symptoms are almost invariably mild; **urethral discharge** (sometimes noticed in the morning only); **urethral pruritis**; or symptoms of any complication. Examination of the urethra shows scanty mucoid (often characteristically grey in colour) or mucopurulent discharge in most cases. Other abnormal findings, apart from a 'two glass' test indicating anterior urethritis, are rare. It is important to remember that trichomoniasis in men is frequently associated with structural abnormalities, such as urethral stricture, and to investigate appropriately whenever the infestation is found.

BACTERIAL VAGINOSIS (BV)

This condition, also known as **anaerobic vaginosis** (**AV**), is the most common diagnosis made in women complaining of abnormal vaginal discharge. The typical symptomatology is complaint of **malodour**, often associated with increased **vaginal discharge**, which is frequently more noticeable after menstruation or coitus. Occasionally, the patient may complain of vulval pruritus or perivulval rash. Examination reveals characteristic increased thin, white or grey-yellow, homogeneous discharge, often containing small bubbles with a characteristic musty/**fishy** odour: mucosal reaction is usually slight. Vaginal pH is >4.5.

Mixing a small amount of vaginal fluid with 10% potassium hydroxide (the **amine test**) often causes the odour to be reproduced due to the release of volatile amines (putrescine, cadaverine).

Microscopy of Gram-stained vaginal exudate shows **'clue cells'** (epithelial cells covered with a large number of Gram-variable coccobacilli) with a small number of polymorphonuclear leucocytes and a decreased number of lactobacilli. Cultures (when performed) show increased numbers of *Gardnerella vaginalis*, ureaplasmas, mycoplasmas, *Mobiluncus* species and anaerobes. These organisms are also frequently found in asymptomatic individuals but in much lower numbers. Thus, there is an imbalance of the normal vaginal flora in BV, with possibly a synergistic relationship between the increased numbers of *G. vaginalis* and anaerobes. Exclusive sexual transmission has not been proved, although the condition is most often diagnosed in sexually active women. Anaerobes as well as *G. vaginalis* (formerly known as *Haemophilus vaginalis* and *Corynebacterium vaginale*) can be found in about 10% of male partners but are not known to be pathogenic in the urethra.

Recent interest has been in the finding that bacterial vaginosis is associated with pregnancy-related complications, such as preterm birth, low birthweight and postabortive and postpartum endometritis.

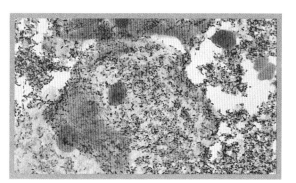

← 283 Clue cells
Note that the epithelial cells are obscured by numerous adherent Gram-variable coccobacilli (***Gardnerella vaginalis***).

Diagnosis
Diagnosis of bacterial vaginosis is made by finding clue cells. Homogeneous grey-white discharge, vaginal pH > 4.5 and positive potassium hydroxide (KOH) test (for volatile amines) are supportive findings.

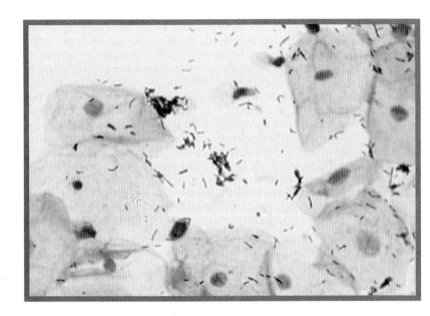

↑ **284 Gram stain of normal vaginal fluid**
showing epithelial cells and lactobacilli.

INTESTINAL PROBLEMS IN MALE HOMOSEXUALS

Some sexual practices in homosexual men facilitate the transmission of pathogenic intestinal organisms. These practices include anal intercourse (both penetrative and receptive), oral intercourse (insertive and receptive), linguoanal contact ('rimming') and some manual practices such as 'fisting' which may also involve foreign objects or trauma.

The diseases that may be found include worm and protozoal infections (e.g. *Giardia lamblia*, *Entamoeba histolytica*), bacterial infections (e.g. *Salmonella*, *Shigella* species, *Campylobacter* species) and NSGIs. In addition, manifestations of the conventional sexually transmitted diseases (syphilis, gonorrhoea, LGV, chlamydia, herpes and warts) that occur in the rectum or anal region are discussed elsewhere in this book. Also, the many intestinal problems associated with HIV infection are discussed in the relevant section.

The conditions may be asymptomatic or present as proctitis or proctocolitis or enteritis with diarrhoea and rectal discharge of mucous, muco-pus; occasionally bloodstained. The exact aetiology is determined by clinical and laboratory examination.

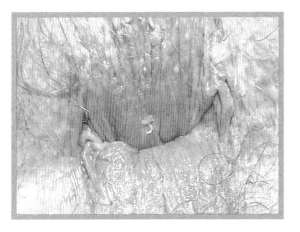

← **285 *Enterobius vermicularis***
at anus.

VIRAL INFECTIONS (EXCLUDING HIV)

HEPATITIS VIRUSES
Several of the viruses which cause hepatitis can be sexually transmitted. It is beyond the scope of this book to describe the clinical presentations in these cases, but brief mention will be made concerning the area of sexual transmission.

Hepatitis A (HAV)
HAV is transmitted by the faeco-oral route and some studies (but not all) have found a higher prevalence of of antibodies in the serum of homosexual men than heterosexual men.

Hepatitis B (HBV)
Although commonly transmitted vertically or parenterally, hepatitis B is quite easily transmitted sexually, as it is often found in high titre in various body fluids. Acquisition of HBV in adult life is often asymptomatic with development of immunity, although a proportion of individuals will become chronic carriers. In some Western countries, over 50% of homosexual men attending STD clinics may have serological markers of hepatitis B infection when there are only very low levels (under 1%) in the general population.

Hepatitis C (HCV)
Although HCV can undoubtedly be sexually transmitted, the predominant route for acquisition is parenteral. It is thus commoner in injecting drug users and those unfortunate enough to have received contaminated blood products. Evidence suggests that sexual transmission is commoner if the source is an individual who has been coinfected with both HIV and HCV. This is perhaps due to a consequent higher copy number of HCV.

Many other viruses that can be sexually transmitted may have a hepatitic component, e.g. Epstein–Barr, cytomegalovirus (CMV), Marburg and HIV.

Herpes genitalis (herpes simplex)

Herpetic lesions are the most common form of genital ulceration in developed countries. Initial infection is frequently followed by recurrent attacks at irregular intervals, often over a period of many years. In the first instance, the infection is usually transmitted sexually (including by orogenital contact) or from other herpetic lesions, e.g. herpetic whitlow. Recurrences are not necessarily related to sexual activity. Overt transmission to sexual partners is seen occasionally: perhaps this is because many adults have herpes antibody (to herpes simplex virus (HSV) 1, HSV 2 or both) in their serum (even in the absence of a history of the condition) and are consequently immune (partially or completely) or have asymptomatic infection. The physical consequences of herpes simplex are usually of little significance. However, the psychological reaction to infection can cause severe problems, and it is essential to discuss the natural history of the disease in detail to help patients achieve a proper perspective.

Severe and persistent recurrences of herpes are common in immunocompromised patients, including those with HIV-related diseases (see p. 321).

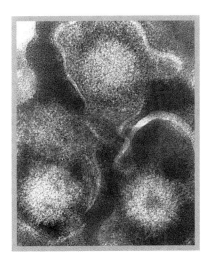

← 286 Electron microphotograph of *Herpes simplex* Type II showing internal capsid and surrounding envelope.

Cause

The virus, **herpes simplex type 2 (HSV 2)**, is responsible for most genital lesions, although **herpes simplex type 1 (HSV 1)** is not uncommon and its prevalence depends on the frequency of orogenital contact. **Herpes zoster** may also cause typical genital lesions. After initial infection, the virus becomes established for life in the nervous system; reactivation with the appearance of clinical lesions may occur from time to time, generally less frequently as the years pass. Usually no pattern for the recrudescence can be determined. Reactivation is less common with HSV 1 than HSV 2.

Clinical course
The incubation period of primary attacks is short, usually between 3 and 6 days. In recurrent attacks, provocation (only occasionally recognized) often causes activity within 1–2 days.

The attack usually begins with the appearance of a group (or groups) of tiny papules which may be pruritic or painful; pruritus may occur at the site of the eruption before the lesions appear. First attacks in adults are often very painful, with large numbers of extensive lesions (occasionally also extragenital), and are associated with mild constitutional disturbance. Severe dysuria is frequent in females and urinary retention may occur due to local symptoms. At times, urinary retention may occur as a consequence of sacral radiculomyelopathy; this may also cause sensation changes and constipation. Primary episodes tend to be less severe in those individuals who have been previously exposed to HSVs. Recurrences are usually less painful or are pruritic only and nearly always occur at the site or sites of initial infection.

Virus is shed from the primary lesions and recurrent lesions for several days after ulceration or erosions first appear: the patient is infectious by contact during the period of virus shedding. Transient virus shedding also occurs in individual with herpes (whether recognized or unrecognized) without any symptoms. This asymptomatic virus shedding is thought to occur in at least 50% of persons with herpes and accounts for many primary episodes in which the source of the infection is not obvious.

Diagnosis
Diagnosis of genital herpes is usually easy, particularly in recurrent attacks, but considerable morphological variation occurs: examination to exclude syphilis is essential.

The virus may be grown in tissue culture inoculated from lesions or detected by a variety of antigen detection tests (ELISA, immunofluorescence) or by electron microscopy. Characteristic changes caused by herpes may be recognised in cervical exfoliative cytology.

Serological tests are of limited value as many patients will have pre-existing HSV antibodies. Type-specific antibody assays are now available and population-based studies show rapidly increasing rates of antibody to HSV 2 after the onset of sexual activity. These studies suggest that the majority of people acquiring infection are probably asymptomatic.

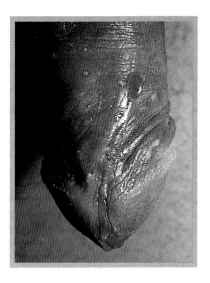

← 287 Herpes simplex
Typical recurrence.

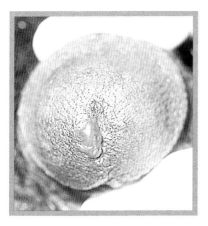

↑ 288 Herpes simplex
Meatal vesicles. Presented as recurrent non-gonococcal urethritis. Vesicles noted on third visit.

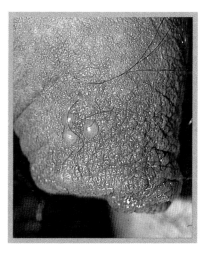

↑ 289 Herpes simplex
Preputial vesicles.

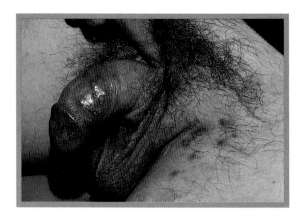

← 290 Primary herpes
Note extensive lesions and tissue reaction.

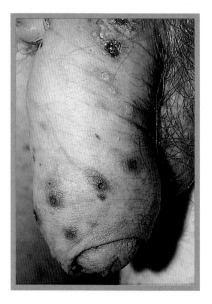

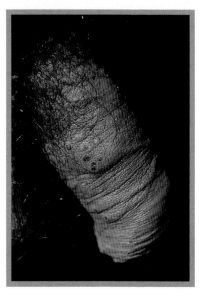

↑291 Herpes simplex
Primary episode, extensive lesions.

↑ 292 Recurrent herpes
Early papular lesions of penile shaft. The oedema surrounding the group of papules is very characteristic: the whole area is usually pruritic.

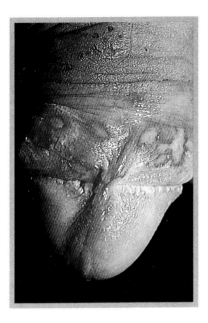

← 293 Recurrent herpes
Healing group of early papular lesions of penile shaft and active erosions of prepuce.

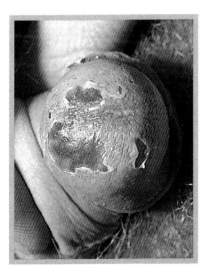

← 294 Recurrent herpes
Superficial erosions (cf. candidiasis, **264**).

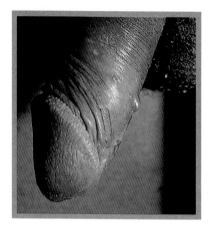

↑ 295 Recurrent herpes
Typical lesions (cf. chancroid, **178**).

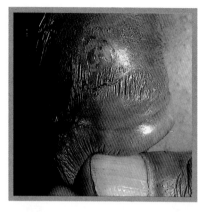

↑ 296 Recurrent herpes
Solitary large erosion of penile shaft
(cf. LGV, **192**).

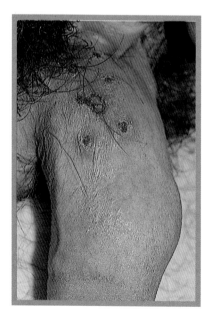

← 297 Recurrent herpes
Lesions on prepuce and penile shaft.

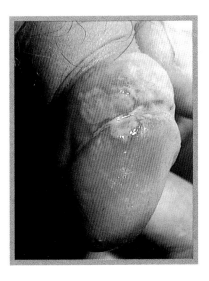

← 298 Recurrent herpes
Herpetic erosions of prepuce, corona and glans penis.

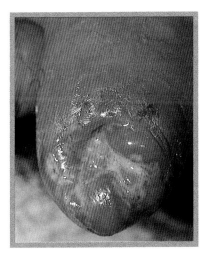

↑ 299 Primary herpes
Phimosis, erosions and balanoposthitis (cf. candidiasis, **266** and primary syphilis, **67**).

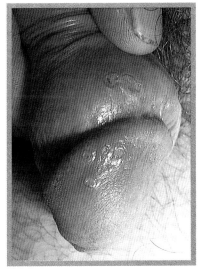

↑ 300 Recurrent herpes
Erosions with marked oedema.

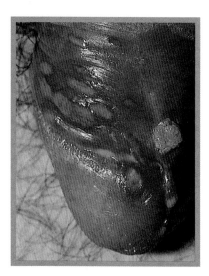

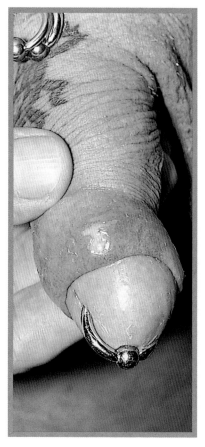

← 301 Recurrent herpes and warts.

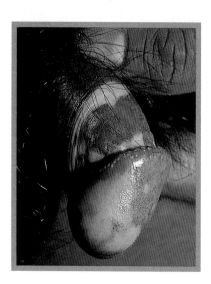

↑ 302 Postherpetic depigmentation (cf. 17).

↑ 303 Herpes and high fashion!.

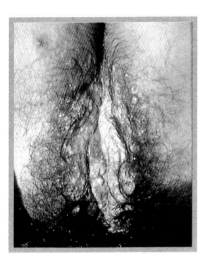

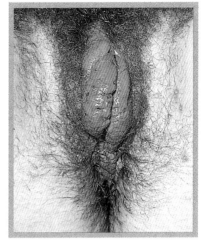

↑ **304 Herpes simplex**
Primary episode showing multiple lesions.

↑ **305 Primary herpes**
Erosions and gross vulval oedema (cf. candidiasis, **255**).

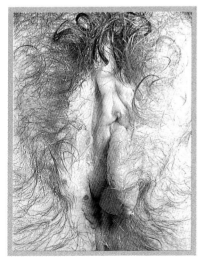

← **306 Herpes simplex**
Primary episode.

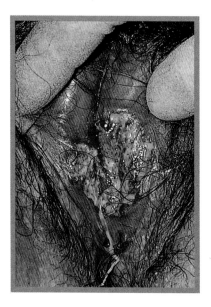

↑ 307 Recurrent herpes
Extensive secondarily infected herpes
of labia.

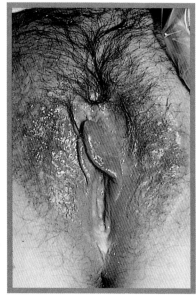

↑ 308 Herpes simplex
Primary episode.

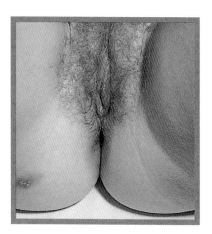

← 309 Recurrent herpes
Herpetic vulvitis and lesions on
buttock.

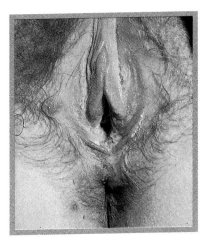

← 310 Recurrent herpes
Note interlabial adhesions.

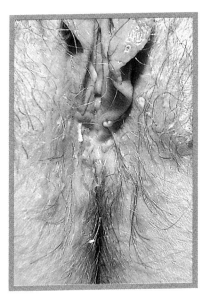

↑ 311 Recurrent herpes
Herpetic erosions of labia, perineum and anus.

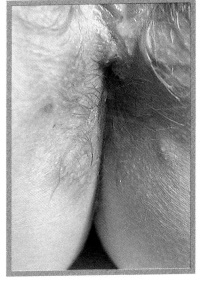

↑ 312 Recurrent herpes
Close-up showing perineal and perianal lesions.

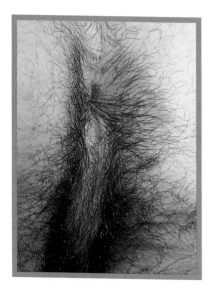

↑ **313 Perianal lesions**
(not HIV positive).

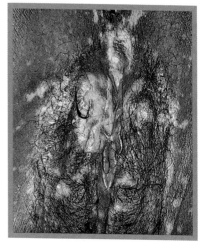

↑ **314 Recurrent herpes**
Vulval herpes, showing active lesions
and depigmentation at sites of
previous lesions.

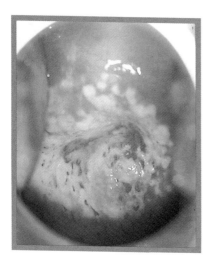

← **315 Primary herpes**
Extensive herpes of cervix.

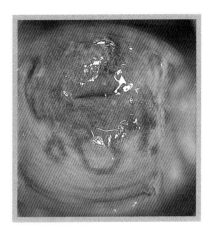

↑ **316 Primary herpes**
Erosions on cervix.

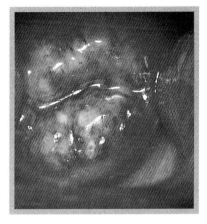

↑ **317 Recurrent herpes**
Active herpes of cervix (cf. **315**).

← **318 Herpes simplex**
Primary lesion on lip. Note
resemblance to primary syphilis (**85**).

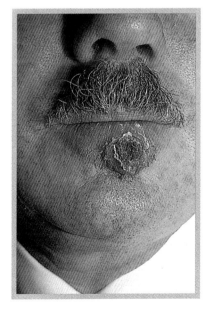

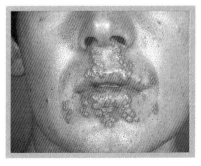

↑ **319 Primary herpes**
Perioral herpes. The patient had
concurrent genital herpes.

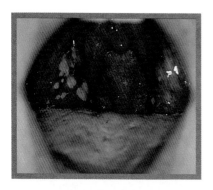

← 320 Primary herpes
Tonsil.

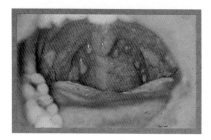

← 321 Primary herpes
Herpetic vesicles on pharynx, with concurrent genital herpes.

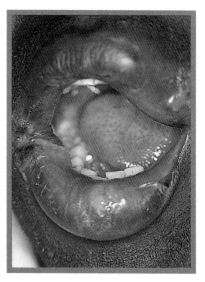

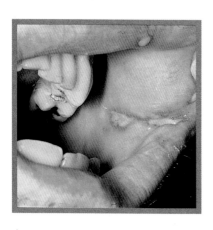

↑ 322 Primary herpes
Buccal lesions.

↑ 323 Recurrent herpes
The patient was HIV-positive.

Herpes zoster

Herpes zoster (**shingles**) occasionally affects the anogenital region. The clinical findings are similar to those in herpes simplex infection, but the symptoms are usually more severe and lesions persist for several weeks. The first manifestation of infection is usually localized hyperaesthesia, followed a few days later by the typical vesicular eruption. Symptoms and signs are almost always unilateral. Recurrence is rare, although localized hyperaesthesia may persist for some time.

In patients with HIV infection, severe herpes zoster (often affecting two or three dermatomes simultaneously) is common (see p. 321).

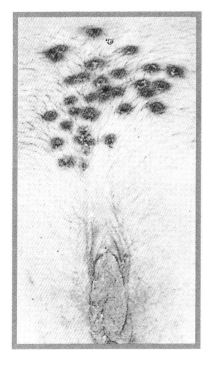

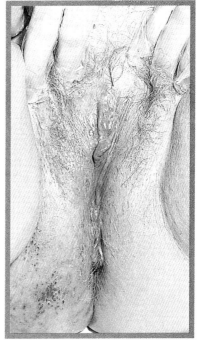

↑ **324 Herpes simplex**
of pubis (for comparison).

↑ **325 Herpes zoster**
Vulva and buttock.

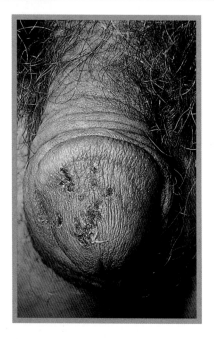

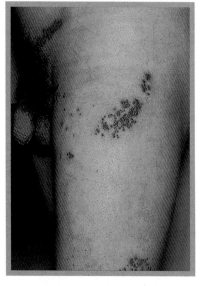

↑ 327 Herpes zoster
Thigh and groin.

↑ 326 Herpes zoster
Penis.

Molluscum contagiosum

This condition is caused by a virus which is transmitted by direct contact, and is a common (usually non-genital) finding in young people. After an incubation period of 2–7 weeks, small, shiny, umbilicated, hemispherical, white papules appear at sites of inoculation. The lesions gradually enlarge, reaching a maximum diameter of 8–10 mm. Molluscs may be found anywhere on the body: in the genital region, they are usually seen on the pubis or penis. Lesions are asymptomatic or slightly pruritic. Occasionally they may become erythematous from excoriation. The condition is usually easily cured.

In patients with HIV infection, there may be numerous lesions, especially on the face; these patients often pose a difficult therapeutic problem (see p. 256).

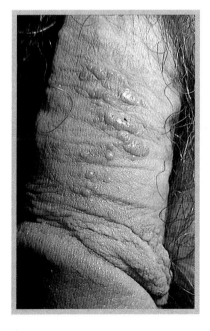

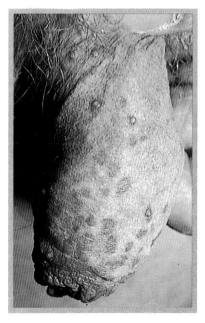

↑ **328 Molluscum contagiosum** of penile shaft and plane warts.

↑ **329 Molluscum contagiosum and lichen planus.**

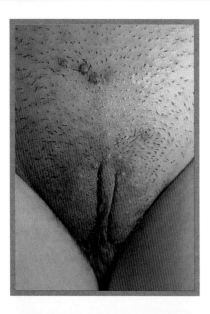

← 330 Molluscum contagiosum of mons. Typical umbilicated lesions.

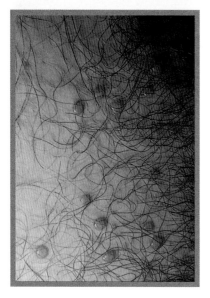

← 331 Molluscum contagiosum of pubis. Typical umbilicated lesions.

Human papillomavirus infection (HPV)
Genital warts

Patients with exophytic genital warts (**condylomata acuminata**) are being recorded in ever-increasing numbers. Although genital warts were previously regarded as banal, research has shown a strong association between wart infections and changes in the cervical epithelium which may progress to **cervical intraepithelial neoplasia** (**CIN**) and later to invasive carcinoma. Similar epithelial changes may occur on the penis (**PIN**), vulva (**VIN**) and at the anus (**AIN**): the significance of these changes is not established.

Warts are caused by the **human papillomavirus** (**HPV**). HPV can certainly be transmitted sexually, but in up to 40% of cases the sexual partner is found to be clear of HPV lesions: in these cases the source of the virus is conjectural. Careful examination of sexual partners of patients presenting with genital warts is essential to reduce the chance of reinfection: examination will often include colposcopy, biopsy, cervical cytology and acetic acid testing.

Warts are occasionally found in infants (more commonly female) in the ano-genital region; rarely they may also be found in the mouth or on the larynx. There is nearly always a history of maternal HPV infection at the time of delivery or in the past: the possibility of child sex abuse should not be overlooked.

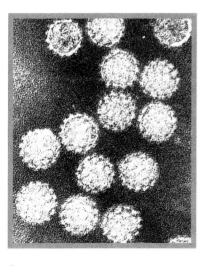

↑ **332 Electron micro-photograph of wart virus.**

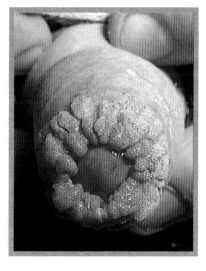

↑ **333 Rosary of warts.**

Human papillomavirus (HPV)

The virus is a member of the **papova** group, and is a DNA virus. There are more than 60 recognized subtypes; types 6, 11, 16 and 18 are particularly linked with genital warts, but there is no practical method (at clinic level) of culturing the virus or determining the subtype.

Clinical course

The incubation period has not been established with certainty. In clinical practice, it is (when determinable) very variable; observation suggests it may sometimes be as little as 3 weeks although research shows it may be up to 1 year. However, many patients with warts have no history of contact with warts; conversely, many partners of patients with warts remain apparently free of infection. Some researchers suggest that most sexually active people acquire HPV, which remains dormant until other (unidentified) factors cause exophytic warts to appear.

The first lesions recognized are usually minute papules or hypochromic areas: the diagnosis, when not clinically obvious, can be established by biopsy. Many of these lesions are so insignificant that they have remained unnoticed by the patient; they are found during examination, usually in the context of attendance as a contact of a known warts case. Overt warts are essentially asymptomatic but the appearance, location, size and the presence of associated conditions are likely to cause attendance. Bleeding from the warts may occur: when located in the urethra, mucoid discharge is often found. Secondary infection may cause offensive odour, irritation and mild discomfort.

The warts begin as small papillomata, usually multiple. Subsequent growth may produce either filiform, hyperplastic or sessile lesions, depending on the anatomical location. In both sexes, warts are found most commonly in areas subject to trauma during sexual activity including, on occasion, the oropharynx. Neoplastic change has been reported, but it must be extremely rare.

In **male patients**, warts are found slightly more frequently in the uncircumcised. Lesions are found most commonly adjacent to the fraenum, on the glans, in the coronal sulcus and inside the urinary meatus. The shaft of the penis is occasionally involved, rectal and anal and perianal warts are often seen, not only in male homosexuals. Growth in the urethra and anus occasionally extends proximally for 1–2 cm. Most warts seen are filiform or hyperplastic; sessile lesions are found on the glans in circumcised patients and on the shaft of the penis.

In **female patients**, warts are seen most often at the fourchette, on the labia (minora and majora), the perineum and in the perianal region. Warts are occasionally found on the vaginal walls, cervix and rectum. Hyperplastic lesions are much more common than sessile lesions. Occasionally, extremely large masses of warts develop, particularly during pregnancy. Cervical cytology is an essential part of the examination.

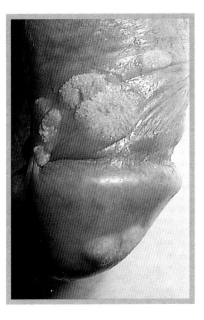

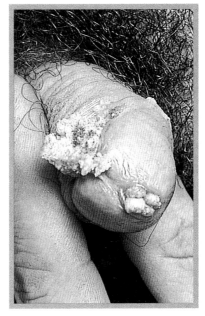

↑ **334 Plane warts**
of prepuce and glans penis.

↑ **335 Meatal and fraenal warts.**
NB: the penis is rotated.

← **336 Warts in coronal sulcus**
A very typical location.

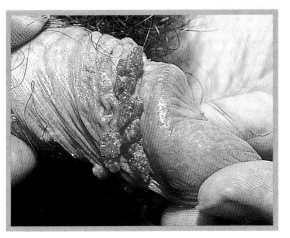

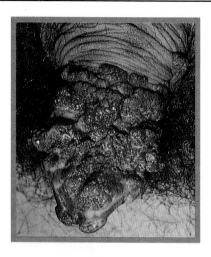

↑ 337 Warts
Exuberant growth.

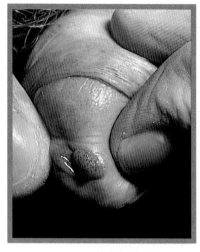

↑ 338 Warts of meatus.

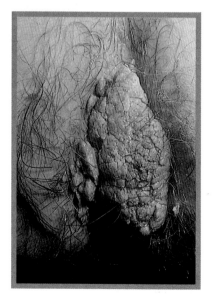

← 339 Massive perianal warts
in male homosexual (cf. **344**).

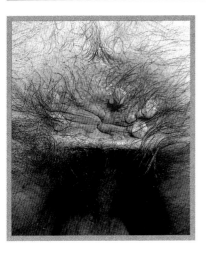

↑ 340 Anal warts
Homosexual patient. Note also fissure.

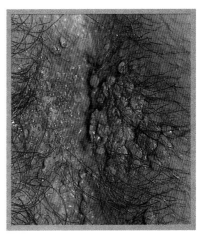

↑ 341 Perianal warts
Extensive lesions.

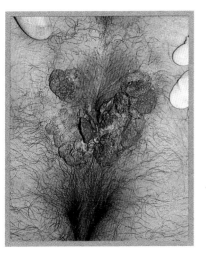

↑ 342 Perianal warts
Lesions presented with bleeding.

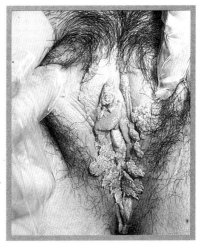

↑ 343 Labial, perineal and perianal warts.

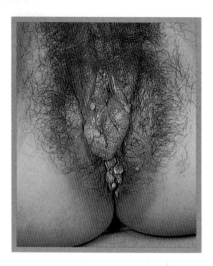

↑ 344 Vulval warts.
The patient also had secondary syphilis which was very difficult to see (cf. **339**)!

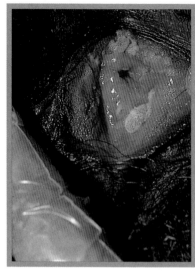

↑ 345 Warts
at introitus.

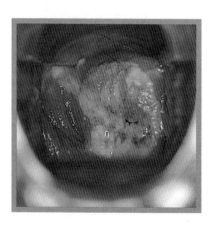

↑ 346 Cervical warts.

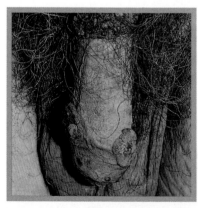

↑ 347 Pigmented papilliform penile lesion
Biopsy was HPV-positive.

Giant condylomata acuminata (Buschke–Lowenstein)

This is an unusual and very rare variety of wart infection. The lesion is a single wart with extensive confluent superficial spread and occasional invasion of underlying tissue. It is reported to be more common on the penis.

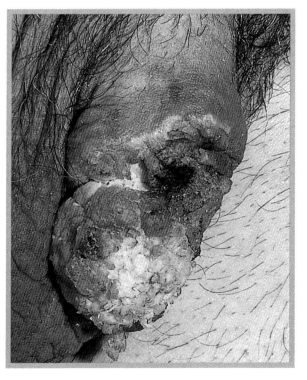

← 348 Giant wart: Buschke–Lowenstein.

OTHER CONDITIONS

BALANOPOSTHITIS

Balanitis (inflammation of the glans penis) and **posthitis** (inflammation of the prepuce) frequently occur concurrently; balanitis alone may occur in the circumcised male but is relatively uncommon. **Balanoposthitis** is seen very frequently, and is often secondary to other conditions. The causes of balanoposthitis are outlined on page 32; many of the conditions listed are discussed separately. Non-specific balanoposthitis is usually mild but can occasionally be severe. Many cases are caused by inadequate hygiene, which is more likely when the prepuce is difficult to retract or when phimosis is present or, conversely, by over-zealous washing, especially with perfumed products. Balanoposthitis may cause discharge and urinary symptoms and is frequently pruritic. Mild cases show diffuse, patchy or generalized erythema with scanty exudate. More severe cases show erosions which may become secondarily infected, and can cause profuse discharge. Occasionally, painful inguinal lymphadenitis is found. Diabetes mellitus may present with balanoposthitis. Routine resting for glycosuria is essential in all cases.

Plasma cell balanitis of Zoon

This is a rare cause of chronic balanitis, usually seen in the middle-aged or elderly. Examination shows one or more superficial red moist shiny plaques with central stippling reminiscent of 'cayenne pepper'. Clinically, the lesion is similar to the premalignant erythroplastic conditions (see p. 233) but is benign. Diagnosis is established by biopsy, which shows characteristic plasma cell infiltration.

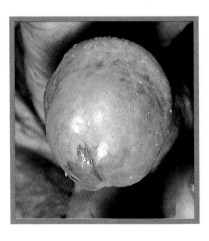

← **349 Mild superficial balanoposthitis.**

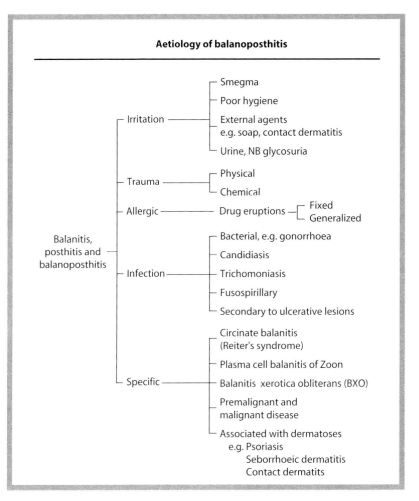

Aetiology of balanoposthitis

Balanitis, posthitis and balanoposthitis
- Irritation
  - Smegma
  - Poor hygiene
  - External agents e.g. soap, contact dermatitis
  - Urine, NB glycosuria
- Trauma
  - Physical
  - Chemical
- Allergic
  - Drug eruptions
    - Fixed
    - Generalized
- Infection
  - Bacterial, e.g. gonorrhoea
  - Candidiasis
  - Trichomoniasis
  - Fusospirillary
  - Secondary to ulcerative lesions
- Specific
  - Circinate balanitis (Reiter's syndrome)
  - Plasma cell balanitis of Zoon
  - Balanitis xerotica obliterans (BXO)
  - Premalignant and malignant disease
  - Associated with dermatoses e.g. Psoriasis Seborrhoeic dermatitis Contact dermatits

↑ **350 Aetiology of balanoposthitis.**

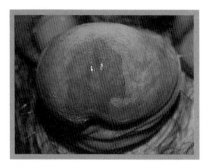

← 351 Plasma cell balanitis of Zoon
Diagnosis established by biopsy.

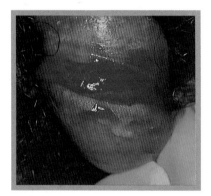

← 352 Plasma cell balanitis of Zoon
The appearance is non-specific; the diagnosis was determined by histology.

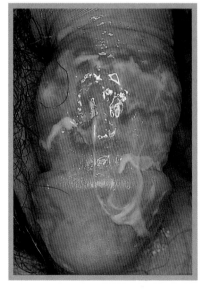

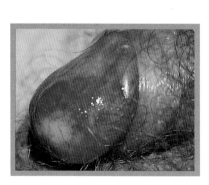

↑ 353 Chronic balanoposthitis
Cause undetermined.

↑ 354 Severe erosive balanitis
Pseudomonas was cultured.

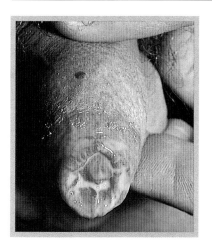

↑ **355 Severe balanoposthitis**
with phimosis and multiple erosions
(cf. candidiasis, **268** and primary
syphilis, **67**).

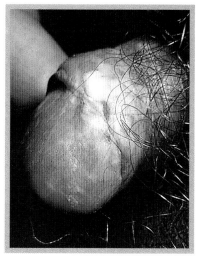

↑ **356 Patchy balanitis**
associated with preputial adhesions.

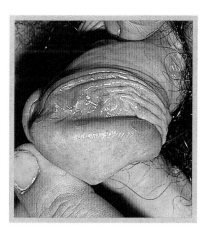

↑ **357 Balanoposthitis**
mainly affecting coronal sulcus.

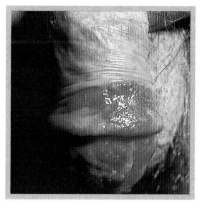

↑ **358 Chronic balanitis**
The patient had mild seborrhoeic
dermatitis.

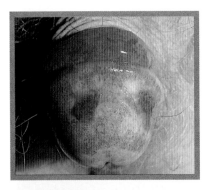

← 359 Balanoposthitis
of uncertain aetiology, lesions on glans and coronal sulcus.

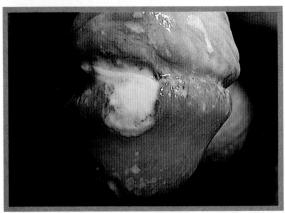

← 360, 361 Ecthyma of glans and prepuce
Note irregular infected ulcerated crusted lesions which healed with minimal scarring.

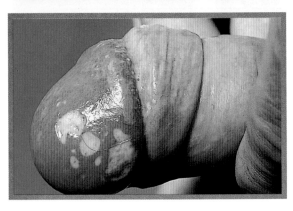

BEHÇETS SYNDROME
Genital aphthosis
The term **genital aphthosis** is unsatisfactory because it has no adequate definition. It is used to include recurrent minute genital erosions, **Lipschütz ulcers** of the vulva and **Behçet's syndrome**, but it is not clear whether these are separate entities or differing manifestations of a common, unknown cause. It seems probable that a proportion of cases diagnosed as genital aphthous ulceration and Lipschütz ulcers in the past were unrecognized **herpes simplex** infections.

Behçet's syndrome (triple syndrome)
Behçet's syndrome is a condition characterized by recurring **genital** and **oral ulceration**, frequently associated with **eye lesions** and **pyoderma** and occasionally, in late stages, with development of neurological, gastrointestinal, cardiac or pulmonary lesions. **Formes frustes** are probably more common than is generally recognized, particularly as the course of the disease may be prolonged. The first manifestation is usually the appearance of morphologically similar ulcers on the genitalia and in the mouth, but lesions may not occur concurrently. The ulcers are usually very painful, 5–20 mm in diameter, with an erythematous halo and have a base covered with yellow slough. Single lesions are most common and scarring from previous lesions may be evident. In male patients the genital ulcer is usually found on the **scrotum** but may occur on the **penis**; in female patients ulceration is usually on the **labium majorum**. Oral lesions occur most commonly inside the **lower lip** but may be found anywhere within the buccal cavity. Ulcerated lesions usually heal in 1–2 weeks but occasionally persist longer. Eye symptoms include **conjunctivitis, uveitis** and **hypopyon**. The interval between relapses frequently exceeds a year and is very variable. The diagnosis is made on a basis of history, physical findings and exclusion of other conditions; there are no pathognomonic investigations.

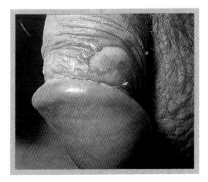

← 362 Behçet's syndrome
Typical penile ulcer. Note erythematous margin.

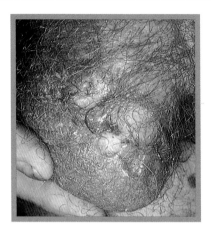

↑ **363 Behçet's syndrome**
Typical scrotal ulceration.

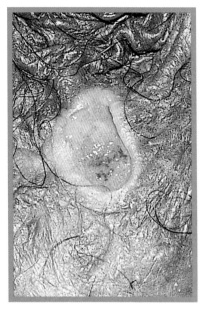

↑ **364 Behçet's syndrome**
Solitary ulcer of scrotum.

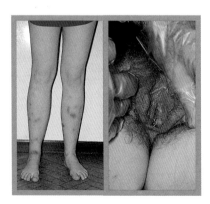

↑ **365 Behçet's syndrome**
Vulval ulcer and erythema nodosum.

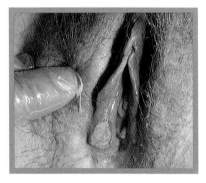

↑ **366 Behçet's syndrome**
Same patient as in **367**. Concurrent ulceration of labium minus.

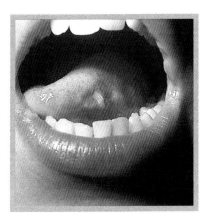

↑ 367 Behçet's syndrome
Lip ulcer and tongue ulcers.

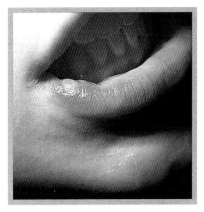

↑ 368 Behçet's syndrome
Lip ulcer. Note scarring from previous episodes.

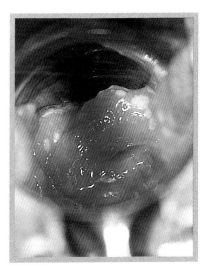

↑369 Behçet's syndrome
Cervix.

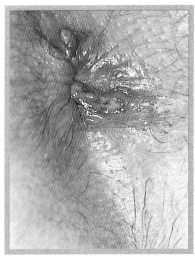

↑ 370 Behçet's syndrome
Perineal ulcers.

ERYTHRASMA

Erythrasma of the groin is a relatively common, unimportant, chronic cutaneous infection. It is seldom the sole reason for attendance and is usually found fortuitously. It is caused by *Corynebacterium minutissimum* which can be demonstrated in stained smears taken from involved areas. Infection commonly occurs in skin folds; in the anogenital area, it may be found on the pubis, scrotum, thigh, groin and natal cleft. Lesions are usually well-defined, pink or brown in colour and dry and scaly. Mild pruritus may occur, but often the condition is asymptomatic. Examination of affected areas under Wood's light shows a characteristic coral-pink fluorescence.

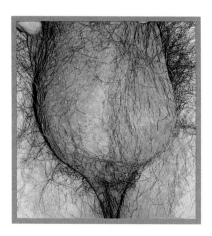

↑ **371 Erythrasma**
of scrotum and thigh.

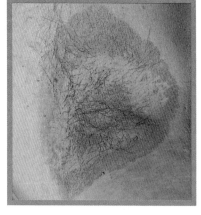

↑ **372 Erythrasma**.
Axilla.

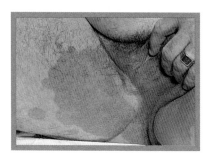

← **373 Erythrasma**
of groin. Cf. with tinea cruris (**378**)
and candidiasis (**272**).

HIDROADENITIS (APOCRINE ACNE)

Apocrine glands in the anogenital area are found in the groin, and in the scrotal, vulval and perianal regions. These glands may be the site of chronic infection which may eventually result in considerable tissue damage. The disease usually begins with discrete, small, subcutaneous nodules which break down to form abscesses that usually later become confluent and discharge on the surface through one or several sinuses. Active lesions and scarring from previous lesions are usually observed. In genitourinary practice, the condition is rare.

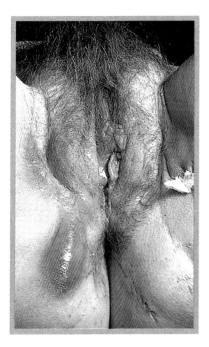

← 374 Hidroadenitis
Note old and active sinuses and evidence of subcutaneous inflammatory lesions.

FUNGAL INFECTIONS

Fungal infections (other than candidiasis, see p. 148) of the anogenital area are common and may affect the penis, groin, scrotum, thigh, vulva or perianal region: males are more frequently affected than females. The lesion on the thigh and scrotum is known as **tinea cruris ('Dhobie itch')**; in many cases, **tinea pedis** can also be found. The diagnosis is established by finding fungal elements in KOH preparations (see p. 57) or by culture. *Epidermophyton floccosum* and *Trichophyton rubrum* are the organisms most often found. The lesion is usually moderately pruritic and spreads slowly. The margin of the area is red and often small satellite lesions are present. Centrally, the involved skin is less erythematous and scaly. Vesiculation occasionally occurs but is rare.

Pityriasis versicolor, caused by *Malassazia furfur*, is another fungal condition that commonly affects the upper parts of the body but may also affect the genitalia. The infection is most common in patients with darkly pigmented skins. Discrete round macules, 1–10 mm in diameter, may be found on the lesions and may become confluent and involve considerable areas. The lesions are a **café-au-lait** colour. Diagnosis is established by mycology.

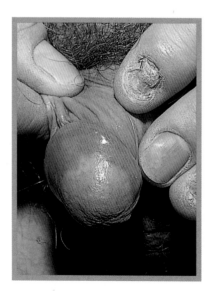

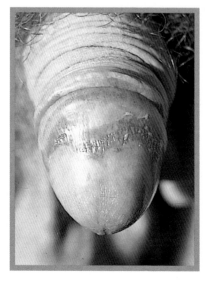

↑ **375 Fungal infection of nail**
Also **psoriasis** of glans and nails.

↑ **376 Fungal infection**
of glans penis.

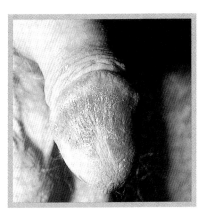

↑ **377 Fungal infection**
of glans penis. Note marginal activity.
Differential diagnosis includes
psoriasis.

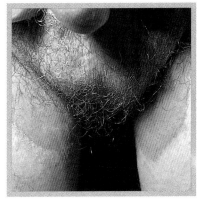

↑ **378 Tinea cruris.**
Typical lesion on thigh (cf.
erythrasma, **372**).

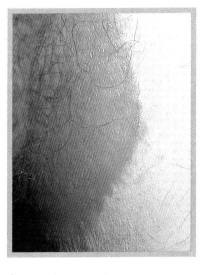

↑ **379 Tinea cruris**
Close-up of edge of lesion showing
satellite follicular lesions.

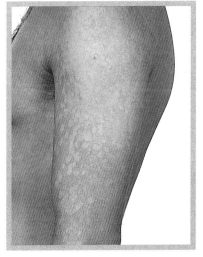

↑ **380 Pityriasis versicolor**
Note morphology and
depigmentation.

LICHEN SIMPLEX

Manifestations of lichen simplex are common in the anogenital region. The condition occurs in predisposed individuals and is usually precipitated by a 'trigger' factor which may be physical or emotional. Severe pruritus ensues and often persists even after the precipitant factor has gone; psychogenic influences are marked. Lesions may be localized or generalized and are often bilaterally symmetrical. Affected areas show lichenification and some oedema: excoriation, fissuring and hyperpigmentation may also be present. Dusky erythema is usual, but red or white areas may also be observed. Lesions may occur anywhere in the anogenital region but are most common on the pubis, vulva (especially in the paraclitoral area), the scrotum and in the groin. There is often a history of failure to improve after treatment with antifungal agents.

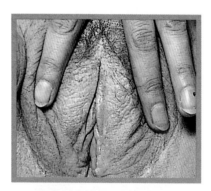

← 381 Lichen simplex
Advanced lesions of vulva and perianal region.

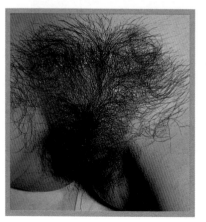

← 382 Lichen simplex (eczema)
This lesion is often aggravated by soap and detergent.

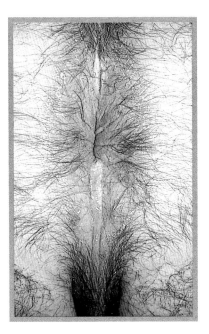

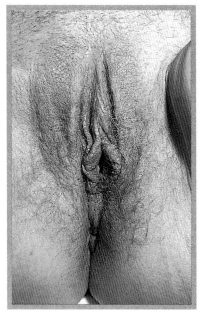

↑ **383 Lichen simplex**
Anus.

↑ **384 Lichen simplex**
Vulva.

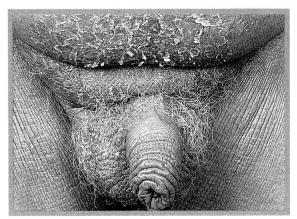

← **385 Lichen simplex**
Severe involvement of pubis, genitalia and thigh.

LICHEN PLANUS

Lichen planus may cause chronic pruritic papular lesions in both males and females. The onset is insidious—patients attend complaining of itchy spots or rash. The lesions are usually papular, 2–15 mm in diameter, sometimes grouped or coalescent. Lesions are usually dusky pink or violaceous in colour but may be white; the surface shows a network of fine lines (**Wickham's striae**). Lesions of lichen planus may be found anywhere on the genitalia; they are most common on the shaft and glans of the penis. In most cases, other manifestations of lichen planus are present: particularly characteristic is the lacy white network on the buccal mucosa of the cheek.

The cause of lichen planus is unknown but psychogenic factors play a considerable part. Lesions usually clear up in less than a year but recurrence occurs in 15–20% of cases.

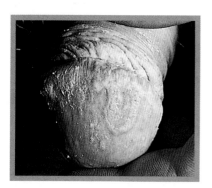

← 386 Lichen planus
Glans penis (same patient as in **387**).

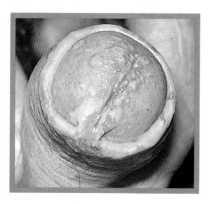

← 387 Lichen planus
Ivory-white lesions on glans penis and prepuce.

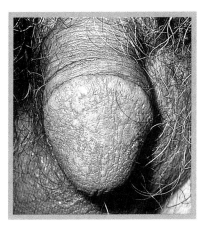

↑ **388 Lichen planus**
Glans.

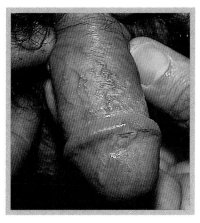

↑ **389 Lichen planus**
Glans penis and shaft.

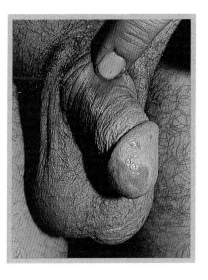

↑ **390 Lichen planus**
'Psoriaform'.

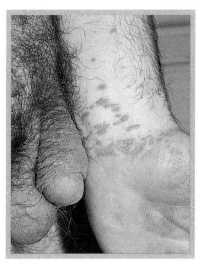

↑ **391 Lichen planus**
Lesions of penis and wrist.

207

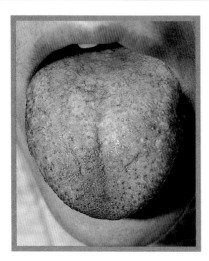

↑ 392 Lichen planus
Tongue.

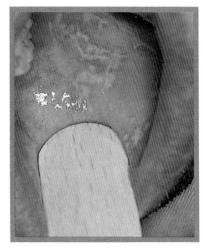

↑ 393 Lichen planus
'Chinese white' patches inside cheek.

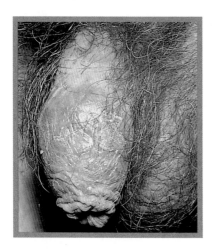

↑ 394 Lichen planus
Extensive lesion on glans penis and scrotum.

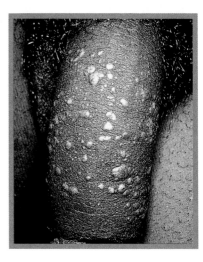

↑ 395 Lichen planus
Chronic lesions on penile shaft.

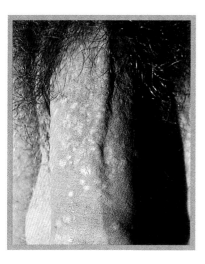

← 396 Lichen planus
Lesions on penile shaft: note active
and healed areas.

Lichen nitidus is thought to be a variant of lichen planus. The condition is
frequently asymptomatic but pruritus may occur. The clinical appearance is
of tiny, white shiny papules, usually multiple and often grouped. Lichen nitidus
is seen most often on the penile shaft. Transient and persistent lesions appear
to be equally common.

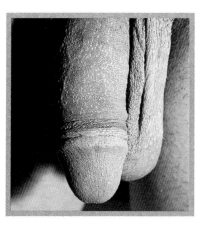

← 397 Lichen nitidus.

PEMPHIGUS VULGARIS

This is an uncommon chronic blistering disease of unknown cause, which occurs more commonly in the middle-aged and in people of Jewish origin. The mucous membranes of the vulva and penis are occasionally involved, usually with evidence of the disease elsewhere on the skin or in the mouth. Bullous and erosive lesions may be found; on mucous membranes, the bullous stage is often transient, and the erosive lesions painful. The lesions on other skin sites are often initially localized. After healing, areas of hyperpigmentation may be found.

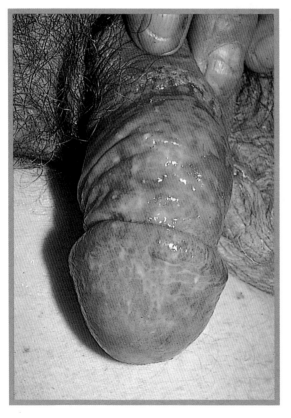

← **398 Pemphigus**
Compare with **265** (candidal balanoposthitis).

PSEUDOACANTHOSIS NIGRICANS

True acanthosis nigricans is associated with malignant disease. A morphologically similar lesion is occasionally seen in obese patients or may occur at puberty. The condition is asymptomatic; examination shows hyperpigmentation and slight lichenification of the vulva, upper thigh and perianal regions. Detailed examination to exclude underlying malignancy should be undertaken: there is no histological distinction between true acanthosis and pseudoacanthosis.

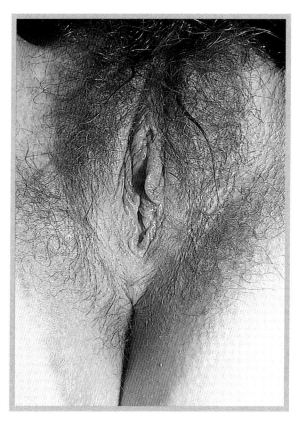

← 399 Pseudo-
acanthosis
nigricans
Marked perianal and
moderate thigh
pigmentation.

PITYRIASIS ROSEA

This condition of unknown aetiology is a classical misdiagnosis for secondary syphilis. The first sign of the disease is the appearance of a **herald patch** which may sometimes occur on the penis but is more often found on the trunk or neck, and occasionally on other sites. The herald patch is a round or oval, bright red, solitary, sharply defined lesion covered with fine scales; the lesion may be 2–4 cm in diameter. The general eruption appears in crops beginning 1–2 weeks after the herald patch. Multiple lesions appear which often follow the lines of cleavage and are commonly found on the trunk and proximal parts of the limbs. The oval or rounded scaly lesions are dull pink at the margin and show central clearing; the size seldom exceeds 1 cm in diameter. Macules are occasionally seen. Pruritus often occurs both in the herald patch and in the general eruption, in contradistinction to the usually non-pruritic secondary syphilis. The eruption clears without residual scarring in 3–6 weeks.

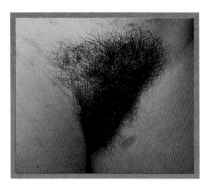

← 400 Pityriasis rosea
Lesions on trunk. Note resemblance to maculopapular secondary syphilide.

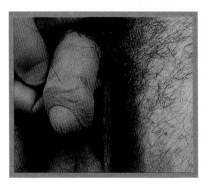

← 401 Pityriasis rosea
Lesions of thigh and penis.

PSORIASIS

Genital lesions are frequently found in this common skin disease of unknown cause. Diagnosis is usually easy because of evidence of psoriasis elsewhere, but genital lesions occasionally occur alone. In many patients with genital psoriasis, typical circumscribed scaly lesions are found, but lesions of the vulva or the glans penis in uncircumcised males may be considerably modified. Lesions in these situations are often non-scaly and diffentiation from other causes of balanitis or vulvitis may be difficult. The lesions are usually bright red and sharply marginated: lichenification (especially in vulval lesions) may be severe. Psoriatic lesions are usually pruritic. The course of the disease is marked by spontaneous remission and relapse.

In patients with HIV infection, severe psoriasis may occur or recur; in these circumstances, control may be difficult (see p. 325).

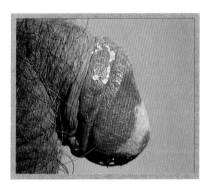

← 402 Psoriasis
of glans penis and prepuce. Note the colour and sharply demarcated margin.

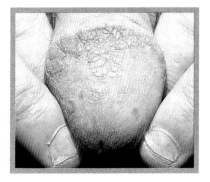

← 403 Psoriasis
of circumcised penis and nails. Note the resemblance of the penile lesion to lichen planus, and also compare with **271**, (candidiasis) and **375**, (fungal infection).

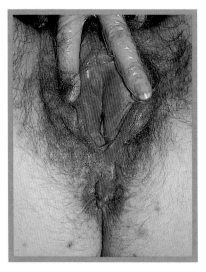

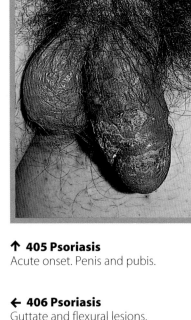

↑ 404 Psoriasis
Lesions on vulva and buttock.

↑ 405 Psoriasis
Acute onset. Penis and pubis.

← 406 Psoriasis
Guttate and flexural lesions.

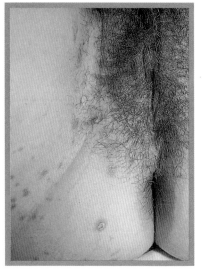

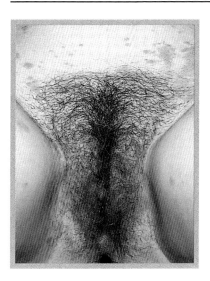

↑ 407 Psoriasis
Abdominal, vulval and thigh lesions.

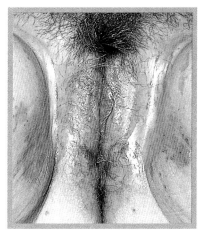

↑ 408 Psoriasis
Flexural lesions with sharply demarcated edges. Compare with **357** (chronic candidal intertrigo).

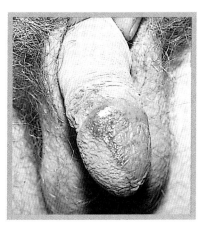

↑ 409 Psoriasis
Penis.

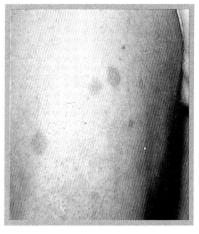

↑ 410 Parapsoriasis en plaque.

SEBORRHOEIC DERMATITIS

Seborrhoic dermatitis is now believed to be a hypersensitivity reaction to abnormally high numbers of normal commensal *Pityosporum* species. The anogenital area is a common site for manifestations in predisposed individuals. Lesions may be found in pubic, crural, vulval and perianal regions. Usually there is evidence of seborrhoeic dermatitis elsewhere on the body, but if anogenital lesions occur alone, differentiation from candidiasis, tinea or psoriasis can be extremely difficult. The lesions are yellowish-red or dull red in colour, diffuse and covered with greasy scales. Chronic lesions may show eczematous change. In flexural sites, the appearance is of intertrigo, often with crusted fissures and secondary infection. Mild to moderate pruritus is common.

In patients with HIV infection, severe exacerbation of seborrhoeic dermatitis affecting the face, chest and other parts of the body is a common clinical problem (see p. 317).

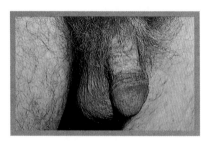

↑ **411 Seborrhoeic dermatitis**
Penis.

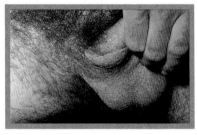

↑ **412 Seborrhoeic dermatitis**
of groin, showing intertrigo and folliculitis.

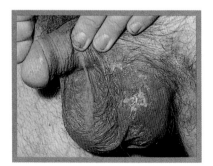

← **413 Seborrhoeic dermatitis**
of thigh and scrotum. Note the yellowish scaling. ***Candida albicans*** was grown on culture but the patient had unequivocal seborrhoeic dermatitis of the chest.

DRUG REACTIONS

Adverse reactions to drugs include toxic effects (which are beyond the scope of this atlas), contact dermatitis (discussed on p. 241) and allergy. Allergic reactions may be either **localized** (**fixed drug eruption**) or **generalized**. The range of drugs that can produce allergic reactions is enormous, but in practice relatively few drugs produce most of the reactions observed. Drug reactions are frequently seen in immunocompromised patients. In this section, common manifestations of drug allergy seen in genitourinary practice are discussed.

Fixed drug eruptions

Fixed drug eruptions often occur in the anogenital region but the reason for this selectivity is unknown. Most lesions seen in practice are caused by sulphonamides, other antibiotics and anti-inflammatory agents. The reaction usually appears shortly after exposure to the allergenic drug as a single (occasionally multiple), well-defined, oedematous or vesicular area, 5–20 mm in diameter, dusky red or brown in colour. The lesion is often extremely pruritic and pigmentary changes may persist for a considerable time. The history of a lesion which reappears in identical form each time a particular drug is used is diagnostic.

Generalized drug reactions

Generalized drug reactions have protean manifestations and the reader is referred to textbooks of dermatology for comprehensive description. From the standpoint of the genitourinary physician, the drugs most commonly seen to cause adverse reactions are penicillin and other antibiotics, barbiturates and anti-inflammatory agents, such as the salicylates and phenylbutazone and related compounds. The types of allergic reaction most frequently observed are urticaria, exanthemata, exfoliative lesions, serum sickness and the Stevens-Johnson syndrome (see p. 247 and 327).

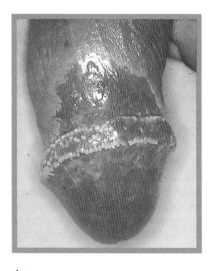

↑ 414 Fixed drug eruption
Penicillin. The lesion simulates
balanoposthitis. Note also **hirsutes
follicularis**.

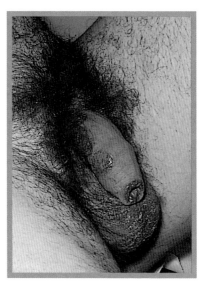

↑ 415 Fixed drug eruption
Sulphonamide.

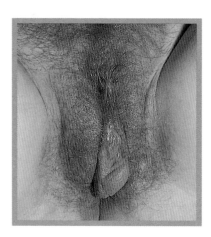

↑ 416 Fixed drug eruption
Sulphonamide.

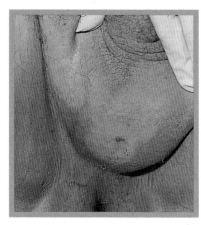

↑ 417 Fixed drug reaction
Erythromycin.

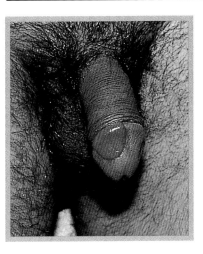

↑ 418 Fixed drug eruption
Sulphonamide (cf. primary syphilis, **62**).

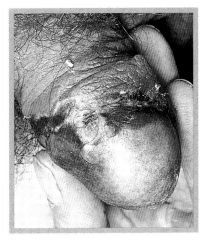

↑ 419 Fixed drug eruption
Barbiturate.

← 420 Fixed drug reaction
Phenylbutazone. Lesions on hands.

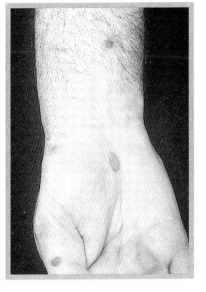

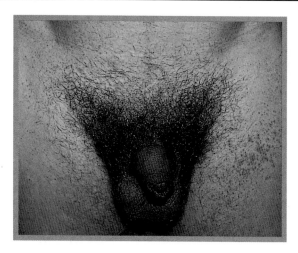

← 421 Drug eruption
Topical nystatin application.

← 422 Generalized drug reaction
Sulphonamide.

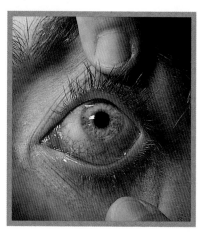

↑ 423 Drug reaction
Tetracycline.

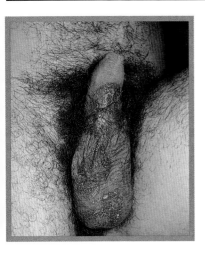

↑ **424 Fixed drug reaction**
Sulphonamide.

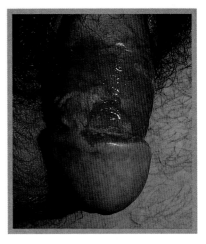

↑ **425 Fixed drug reaction**
Tetracycline.

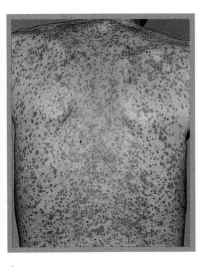

↑ **426 Generalized drug
eruption**
Sulphonamide/diaminopyrimidine.

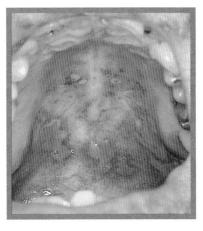

↑ **427 Generalized drug
eruption**
Same patient as **426**. Cf. erythema
multiforme (**488**).

DYSTROPHIC CONDITIONS

There is considerable controversy concerning the relationship of morphologically similar lesions variously labelled **kraurosis, leukoplakia, primary vulval atrophy** and **lichen sclerosus et atrophicus (LS)**. **Balanitis xerotica obliterans (BXO)** is thought to be the equivalent in male patients of LS. Many authorities think that LS is the common underlying condition for patients with dystrophic lesions. LS affects both glabrous and hairy surfaces; primary vulval atrophy affects hairy surfaces only. The cause of both conditions is unknown.

Lichen sclerosus (LS)

LS is a rare generalized skin disease; it is much more commonly localized to the genitalia. It may occur in both males and females. Genital lesions in women are found most frequently in middle age but are not uncommon in younger and older age-groups. Some 30–40% of women with vulval lesions have evidence of the disease in other areas. Vulval lesions may be asymptomatic, but are usually pruritic, or may present with dyspareunia caused by vulval atrophy. In the early stages, patchy pallor is found, most often adjacent to the clitoris or on the perineum: these areas often become normal to the naked eye after treatment. Later, the pallor may become more extensive to involve the perivulval and perianal epithelium; hyperkeratosis and telangiectasia are often seen. Progression is irregular but eventually the whole of the vulva and the anal and perianal regions may be involved; rarely, malignant change may occur. In advanced cases, the dermis is pale, thin and atrophic. Similar anal and perianal lesions may be seen in male patients. When genital lesions are found, evidence of the disease should be sought in other areas, particularly the upper trunk, neck and axillae. Lesions in these situations are slightly raised, flat white macules or papules, often grouped, usually pruritic.

Balanitis xerotica obliterans (BXO)

BXO is the term given to the more severe forms of LS with phimosis, loss of anatomical definition and terminal urethral stenosis, occasionally leading to meatal occlusion. Many patients remain asymptomatic for a long time. Malignant change has been reported. The condition frequently begins in childhood.

In uncircumcised patients, pale, fibrotic areas are found at the preputial margin and glans penis. Lesions are often initially macular, and as the condition progresses, phimosis, recurrent fissuring of the prepuce and adhesion of the prepuce to the glans may occur; many patients eventually require referral for circumcision. Lesions on the glans are similar to those seen in circumcised patients.

In circumcised patients, localized pallid areas with diffuse margins are seen on the glans, more commonly on the ventral surface. In early cases, lesions may be erythematous. Telangiectases may occur in or at the margin of affected areas and bleeding occasionally occurs. In some patients, the fibrosis is confined to the perimeatal region, resulting in meatal narrowing (stenosis). In others, there is fibrosis of the distal urethra and stricture formation: surgical intervention is often necessary. Patients with meatal stenosis may present as cases of NGU.

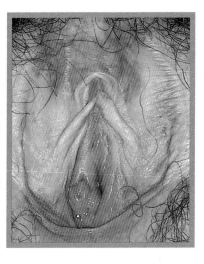

← 428 Lichen sclerosus (LS)
Advanced vulval lesion.

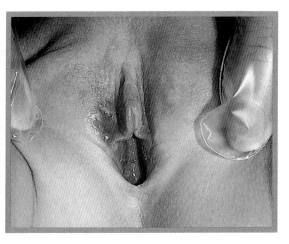

← 429 Lichen sclerosus
Patient was 10 years old.

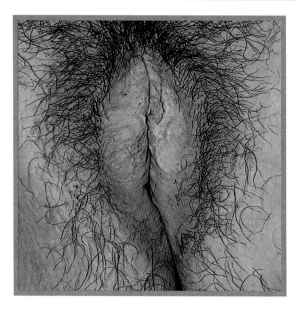

← 430 Lichen sclerosus
Vulva. The patient presented with 'untreatable thrush'.

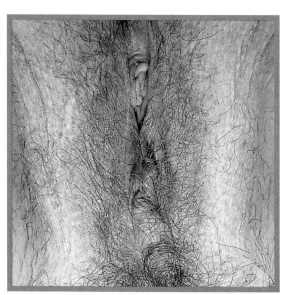

← 431 Lichen sclerosus
Vulval atrophy. Note minute telangiectases.

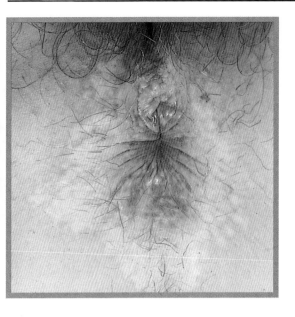

← 432 Lichen sclerosus
Perianal lesion.

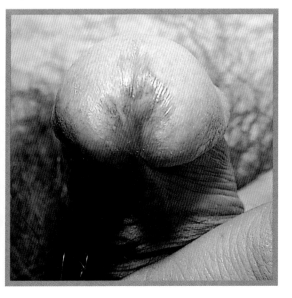

← 433 Balanitis xerotica obliterans (BXO)
Perimeatal atrophy and telangiectasia.

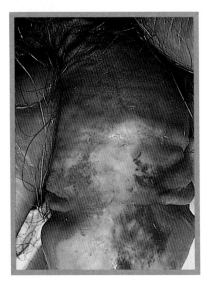

↑ 434 Balanitis xerotica obliterans
Lesions of glans penis, coronal sulcus and prepuce.

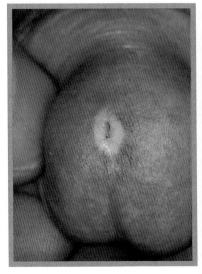

↑ 435 Balanitis xerotica obliterans
Meatal stenosis.

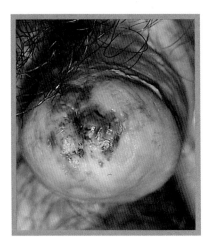

← 436 Balanitis xerotica obliterans
Note pallor and telangiectasia.

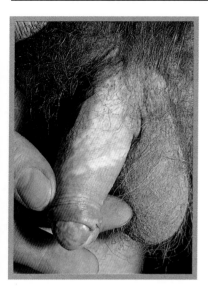

← 437 Balanitis xerotica obliterans
Extensive lesions of shaft and glans penis; prepuce is also affected.

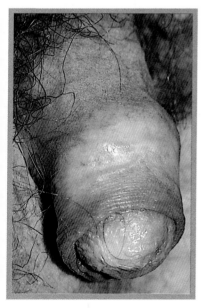

← 438 Balanitis xerotica obliterans: phimosis
Note pallor of glans. This type of case is likely to require circumcision.

PARASITIC INFESTATIONS
Pediculosis pubis

Pubic lice (*Phthirus pubis*, **crabs**) are commonly transmitted during sexual contact, but may also be acquired from infected fomites such as shed hairs, clothing or towels. The lice feed on the skin surface and intense pruritus is produced at the sites of bites. The lice and their eggs (**nits**) are found on hairy locations, such as the pubis, perineum, buttocks and upper thighs; occasionally, they are found in the axillae and rarely on the eyelashes. Crab lice live for about 4 weeks. The female lays 8–10 eggs daily which hatch in about 8 days. Maturity is reached in a further week.

The patient may become aware of infestation because of itching or by noticing movement of the small (1–2 mm) yellow-brown or grey lice, or by finding the minute black or dark-brown nits attached to the base of a hair.

Occasionally, the first evidence of infestation is the appearance of pinhead-sized blood spots on the underwear. Excoriation and secondary infection of affected areas is common. The diagnosis is made by recognition of the louse or nit.

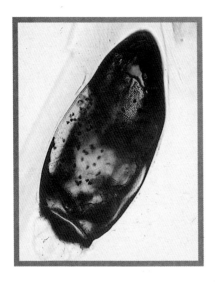

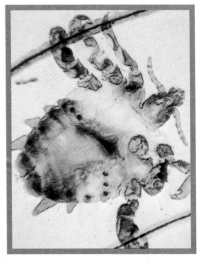

↑ **439 Pediculosis**
Nit containing larva attached to hair.

↑ **440 Pediculosis**
Adult louse attached to hair.

It is worth remembering that parasitophobia is not uncommon: definite evidence of infestation should be sought before treatment is given. A self-inflicted hazard of louse infestation is the severe dermatitis that can be caused by mercury-containing ointments which are traditionally used in treatment (see **479**).

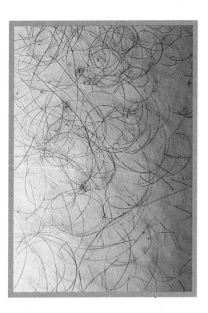

← 441 Pediculosis
Close-up view showing lice and nits on pubis.

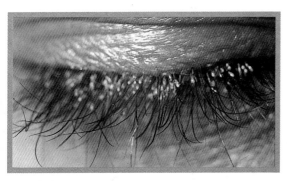

← 442
Pediculosis.
Nits attached to eyelashes.

Scabies

The mite *Sarcoptes scabiei* is frequently transmitted during sexual contact, producing characteristic genital lesions. The lesions may be found anywhere on the genitalia and are also frequently found on the abdomen, wrist, hand and elbow; occasionally other locations may be infested but the face is spared. The lesions are intensely pruritic and, characteristically, pruritus is exacerbated at night or when the patient is warm, e.g. after bathing.

The life of the mite is about 3 weeks. After hatching in a burrow the larvae migrate to a skin pocket and moult several times: maturity is reached in about 2 weeks. The mature mite burrows into the stratum corneum, advancing 1–2 mm daily. The female mite lays two or three eggs daily which hatch in 3–4 days.

The classical clinical lesion is a slightly raised sinuous burrow, which is most often readily identified between the fingers. At other sites, excoriation, secondary infection or eczematous change may distort the appearance. Lesions on the penis and scrotum are frequently oedematous, and lesions in infants may be vesicular.

Diagnosis is usually based on the history and findings: mites can sometimes be extracted from burrows and recognized.

A particularly severe form of scabies, crusted scabies, may be seen in immunocompromised individuals such as those with HIV (see **511–514**).

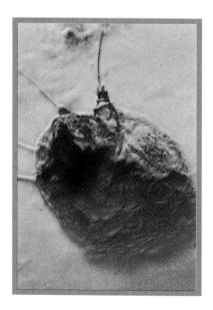

←443 Scabies
Adult *Sarcoptes scabiei* (microscopic view).

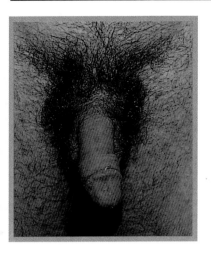

↑ 444 Scabies
Typical extensive scabies of penis, thighs and abdomen.

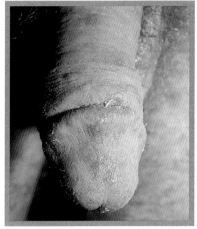

↑ 445 Scabies
Lesions on glans penis. Close-up of lesions in **444**.

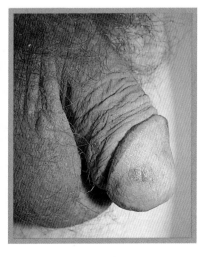

↑ 446 Scabies
Penis and scrotum.

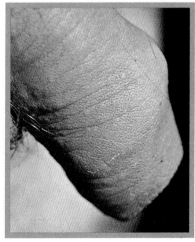

↑ 447 Scabies.
Burrow on penis.

231

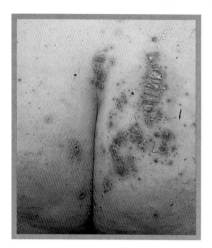

↑ 448 Scabies
Buttock.

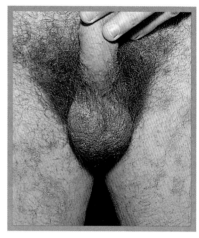

↑ 449 Scabies
Eczematized lesions.

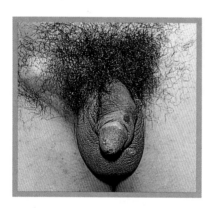

↑ 450 Scabies
Secondarily infected scabies with
inguinal bubo. Note typical
oedematous lesions on scrotum and
penis. The bleeding lesion on the
prepuce was scarified for preparation
of dark-ground specimens.

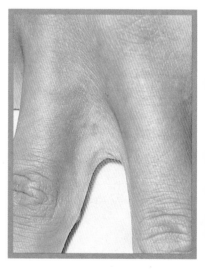

↑ 451 Scabies
Interdigital burrows.

PREMALIGNANT AND MALIGNANT CONDITIONS

Premalignant and malignant conditions occasionally occur in genitourinary practice but are rare. **Erythroplasia of Queyrat**, **Bowen's disease**, **Paget's disease**, **basal cell** and **squamous cell carcinomata** and other neoplasms may be found in the anogenital regions. Reticuloses or secondary deposits may involve inguinal lymph glands. In advanced cases, the diagnosis of malignant disease is usually obvious but early stages may present as lesions simulating balanitis or vulvitis or as genital ulcers. Clinical differentiation is usually impossible and the diagnosis has to be established by biopsy.

In HIV, Kaposi's sarcoma is relatively common on the penis.

Erythroplasia of Queyrat

This premalignant condition may be found on the penis (particularly in uncircumcised patients) or on the vulva. Examination shows a slightly elevated plaque, sharply demarcated with a bright red, clean, velvety surface. The lesion spreads slowly.

Bowen's disease

This intraepidermal carcinoma may be associated with systemic malignant disease. Lesions are found on the penis (frequently in association with chronic balanoposthitis) or vulva. Examination shows a non-elevated plaque with an irregular margin: the lesion has a dark red, crusted or scaly surface. Pruritus of the patch is frequent, and the lesion spreads slowly.

Paget's disease

This intraepithelial carcinoma is frequently associated with an underlying carcinoma and it has been suggested that the surface lesion is a secondary growth. Lesions may be found on the vulva and perianal regions and occasionally on the penis. Examination shows a circumscribed scaly and crusted erythematous plaque, sometimes ulcerated and oozing blood. The lesion is often pruritic.

Melanoma occasionally occur on the genitalia. The lesion is usually slightly raised with irregular margins; it is characteristically hyperpigmented. Biopsy of suspicious lesions is essential.

Penile intraepithelial neoplasia (PIN) and vulval intraepithelial neoplasia (VIN)

These two conditions have recently caused considerable interest. The lesions are discussed in the section of genital warts (see p.185).

Kaposi's sarcoma, lymphoma

These are discussed under HIV (see pp. 291, 297).

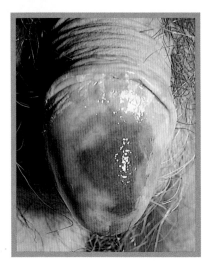

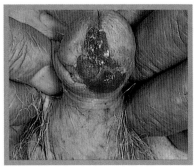

↑ 453 Erythroplasia of Queyrat
Typical lesion. Diagnosis made at biopsy, Zoon was excluded.

↑ 452 Erythroplasia of Queyrat
Lesion showing typical colour, surface and margin.

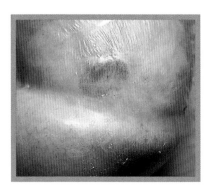

← 454 Erythroplasia of Queyrat
Early lesion.

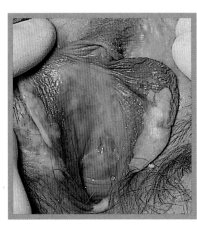

→ 455 Bowen's disease
Note irregular margin and lack of elevation.

Basal cell carcinoma (epithelioma, rodent ulcer)

Basal cell carcinoma is much less common than squamous cell growths. Typical 'rodent ulcers' with a pearly, firm, rolled edge are most often found on the penis: they are rare in other genital areas. 'Chimney sweep's cancer' (epithelioma of the scrotum), an occupational hazard, is now very uncommon.

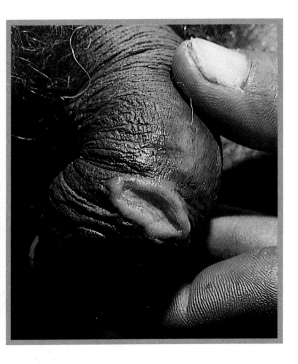

↑ **456 Epithelioma of penis (basal cell carcinoma)**
Note typical rolled edge.

Squamous cell carcinoma

This condition usually develops after middle age and is most common in uncircumcised males. Attendance is often delayed because the lesion is painless. It may present as a warty growth or as an indurated ulcer with a firm edge. Spread is often rapid and involvement of inguinal lymph nodes is frequent. Growths arising from urethral epithelium may present as lumps in the penis, urethral discharge or urinary obstruction.

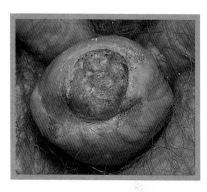

↑ **457 Squamous cell carcinoma.**

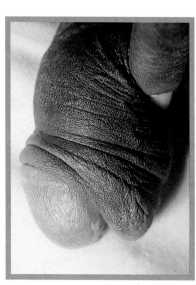

↑ **458 Carcinoma of penis**
Origin unknown. The patient presented as Peyronie's disease and the condition remained unchanged for 2 years. The true diagnosis was established after spread to inguinal nodes and biopsy.

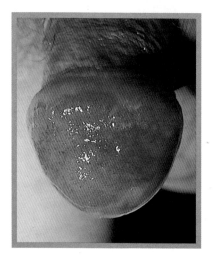

← **459 Squamous cell carcinoma**
Warty lesion.

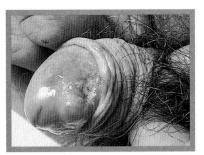

← 460 Squamous cell carcinoma
Ulcerated lesion.

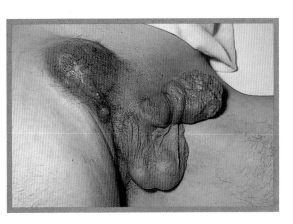

← 461 Advanced squamous cell carcinoma

with secondary deposits in the inguinal glands. The patient was aged 42 years and presented with anxiety that he had a venereal disease. Symptoms had been present for one year.

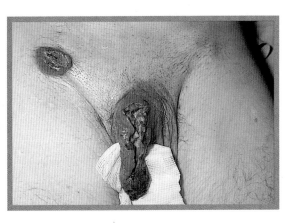

← 462 Squamous cell carcinoma

with almost complete destruction of the penis and fungating secondary deposits. The patient was aged 72 years and referred as '?primary syphilis'.

PYOGENIC LESIONS

The anogenital region, in common with all areas of the body, may be the site of pyogenic skin infections, whose appearance may arouse fears of sexually transmitted diseases. Skin infections are particularly prone to occur in the area for anatomical reasons: hairy skin flexures, numerous glandular structures and proximity to the anus. Septic penile lesions may cause gross local oedema, and adhesions between the prepuce and glans penis are likely to form pockets where infection can readily occur. **Follicullitis, furunculosis, abscess** and **ecthyma** may be found. Most infections are caused by **staphylococci** or **streptococci**. Severe tissue destruction may occur (Fournier, Melaney, necrotisisng fasciitis); several pathogens have been implicated, often in synergy.

In patients with HIV infection, immunodeficiency increases the likelihood of such infections (genital and/or generalized).

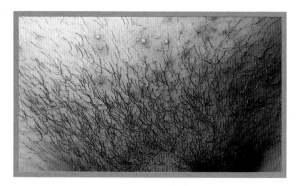

← 463 Pubic folliculitis
Care must be taken to exclude parasitic infestations.

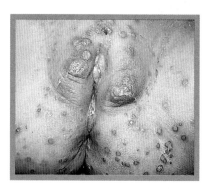

← 464 Napkin rash
Can be confused with congenital syphilis.

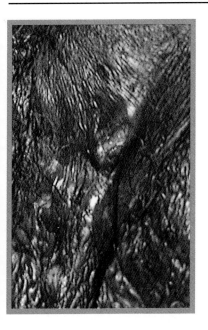

↑ 465 Scrotal folliculitis
Compare with **496** (leprosy).

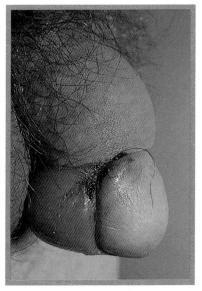

↑ 466 'Saxophone' penis
Marked oedema associated with
minor pyogenic infection. Cf. **72**.

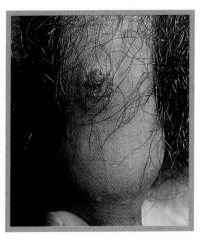

← 467 Penile abscess
Note oedema and erythema.

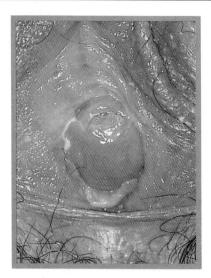

← **468 Para-urethral abscess**

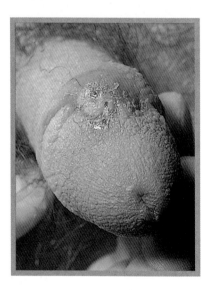

↑ **469 Abscess in coronal sulcus**
Note adhesions.

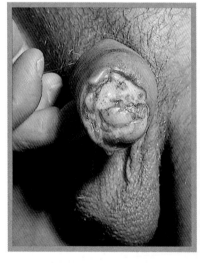

↑ **470 Gangrene of penis**
Fusospirillary infection, showing
marked tissue damage.

TRAUMA

Traumatic lesions of the genitalia from physical damage are extremely diverse: the morphology is variable but history is usually diagnostic. Genital injury may occur during sexual intercourse or masturbation and is sometimes a feature of psychiatric illness. Bizarre sexual practices can result in bizarre physical lesions.

Drugs, disinfectants and other agents may act as irritants when in contact with the skin or mucous membranes of the genitalia in susceptible individuals and may cause **contact dermatitis**. The history is often diagnostic but patients may be reluctant to disclose the truth when the agent has been self-administered. Antiseptics, such as phenolic compounds or potassium permanganate, may be self-applied with prophylaxis against venereal disease in mind. Contact dermatitis may also be provoked by clothing or cosmetics; intravaginal contraceptive tablets, condoms and vaginal diaphragms are other occasional causes. The clinical findings are very variable and include pruritus, erythema, lichenification and, rarely vesiculation. When a specific agent is suspected of causing contact dermatitis patch testing may be helpful.

Therapeutic measures (particularly radiation therapy) may result in lesions which can be termed traumatic.

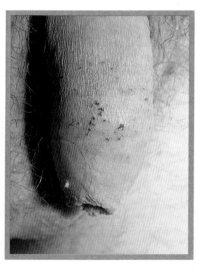

↑ **471 Teeth marks**
after fellatio.

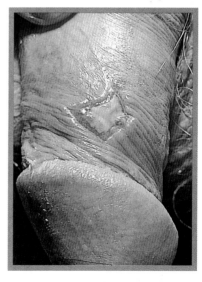

↑ **472 Penile abrasion.**

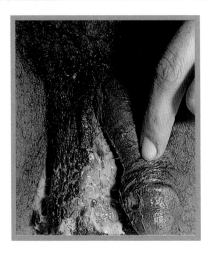

← 473 Severe reaction to podophyllin ointment
which was left on the skin overnight.

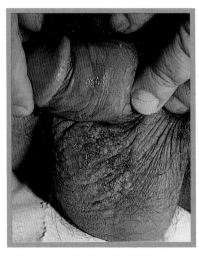

↑ 474 Damage caused by podophyllin ointment.

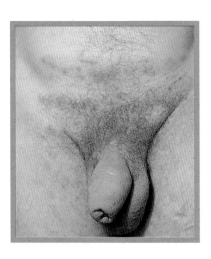

↑ 475 Allergic contact dermatitis
caused by elastic in underwear.

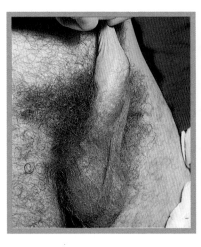

↑ 476 Penile and scrotal contact dermatitis
caused by use of vaginal deodorant.

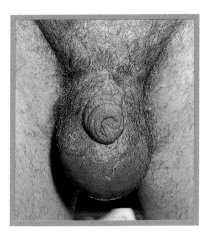

↑ **477. Penile and scrotal contact dermatitis**
caused by use of a detergent containing enzymes.

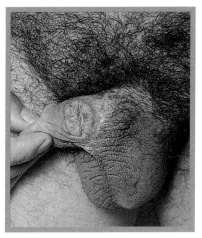

↑ **478 Dermatitis artefacta**
Bizarre lesions are often due to self-inflicted damage.

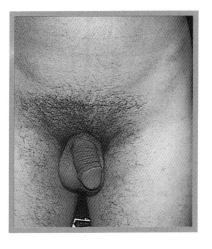

↑ **479 Contact dermatitis**
caused by mercury ointment. Note the characteristic colour.

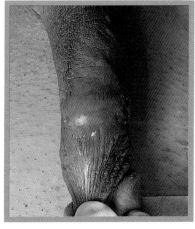

↑ **480. Phenolic disinfectant reaction**
The patient had herpes simplex.

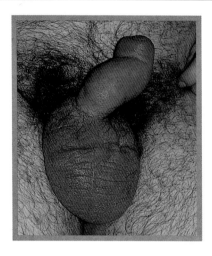

↑ **481 Contact dermatitis**
from condom.

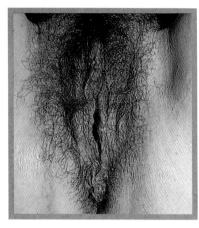

↑ **482 Vulvitis**
caused by phenolic disinfectant
which was diluted 1:2 only.

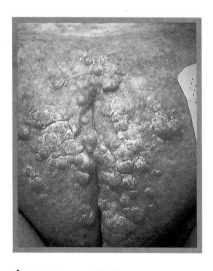

↑ **483 Postradiation
lymphangiectasis**
of pubis.

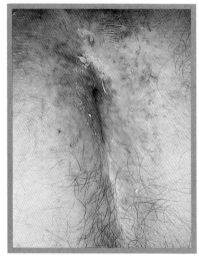

↑ **484 Postradiation dermatitis**
of perianal region.

MISCELLANEOUS
Peyronie's disease

The cause of this condition is unknown, but there is an association with the lesion known as Dupuytren's contracture. Fibrous nodules appear in the corpora cavernosa. The nodules are usually noticed accidentally, but occasionally complaint of deviation of erection (**chordee**) is made. The painless nodules may be single or multiple and vary from pea-size to grape-size; occasionally nodules are confluent. The fibrotic masses may enlarge or regress but the factors which influence change are not known.

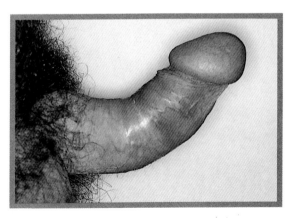

← 485 Plaque of Peyronie's disease

near base of penis. Curvature of the erect penis (chordee) is demonstrated.

Tuberculosis

Cutaneous genital tuberculosis is now extremely rare. The diagnosis is usually established with difficulty by bacteriological or histological methods. The disease may present as chronic painful ulcerative lesions of the penis or vulva (**tuberculosis chancre**) or as a '**cold abscess**' of the groin. Rarely, visceral tuberculosis may present as chronic salpingitis (PID), chronic epididymitis or chronic urinary tract infection. Investigation for *Mycobacterium tuberculosis* is worthwhile in patients with particularly persistent NGU as a small proportion of cases (>1%) are found to be caused by this organism. Sexual transmission is said to occur.

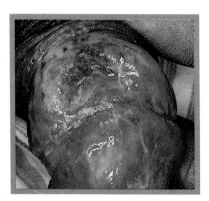

← 486 Tuberculous subpreputial ulcer
Diagnosis was established by biopsy.

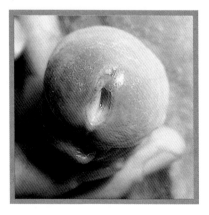

← 487 Tuberculous ulcer of the meatus
The diagnosis was established bacteriologically.

Stevens–Johnson syndrome (erythema multiforme)

The exact aetiology of this condition is unknown, but in about 50% of cases there appear to be antecedent factors which include drug sensitivity and various infections, such as herpes, syphilis and lymphogranuloma venereum. Manifestations follow the precipitant (if present) after an interval of 1–3 weeks. All cases show haemorrhagic bullous and erosive lesions of mucous membranes which affect the penis, vulva and conjunctivae. Stomatitis is usually severe and characteristically causes haemorrhagic crusting of the lips. The genital lesions may simulate balanoposthitis or vulvovaginitis: if the urethra is involved, NGU is often found. Conjunctivitis occurs in most cases and may be complicated by corneal ulceration. Most cases show a skin rash with characteristic 'target' lesions (cyanotic centrally, erythematous at periphery) occurring in crops and principally affecting the extremities. Considerable systemic disturbance and fever are common. Diagnosis is made on clinical grounds; complete recovery occurs after 2–3 weeks.

Erythema multiforme is not uncommon in HIV (see **632**).

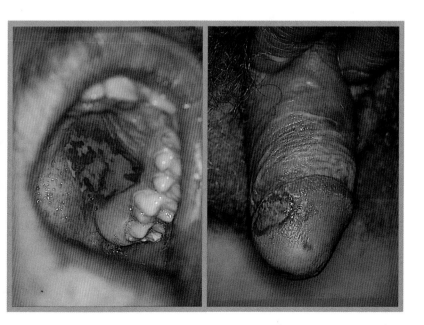

↑ **488 Erythema multiforme**
Lesions of penis and palate.

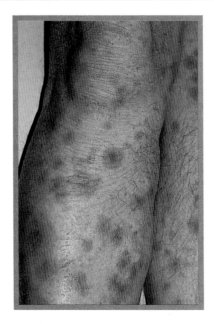

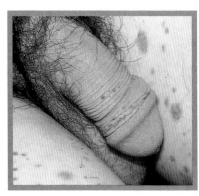

← 489 Erythema multiforme
Typical 'target' lesion.

↑ 490. Erythema multiforme
Lesions on penis and thigh.

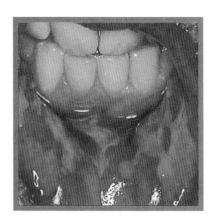

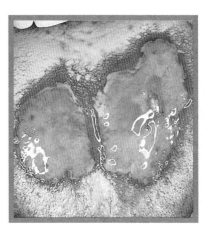

↑ 491 Erythema multiforme
Stomatitis. Note the crusted blood on the lips.

↑ 492 Erythema multiforme
Lesions of tongue.

Crohn's disease

This condition, also known as **regional ileitis**, is an intestinal disease of unknown aetiology. The rectum and anus are often involved at an early stage by the development of perianal and perirectal abscesses. These commonly form fistulae on the skin adjacent to the rectum; genital lesions are rare. The fistula may appear to be a granulomatous ulcer and, as such, may provoke attendance, particularly in anoreceptive homosexuals. The diagnosis is usually established by the history of intestinal disorder, radiological investigation and by biopsy of the superficial lesion. The ulcer is frequently painless and may be the sole manifestation present.

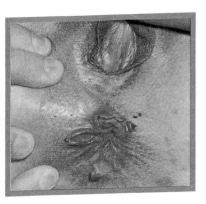

← 493 Crohn's disease
Perianal ulceration, sometimes the presenting manifestation. Note the similarity to anal primary syphilis.

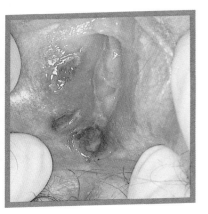

← 494 Crohn's disease
Vulval lesion.

Cutaneous amyloidosis

This rare condition of unknown cause has several different clinical patterns: the diagnosis is usually established by biopsy. Localized tumours may occur anywhere on the skin surface and the lesion is usually asymptomatic. Diffuse infiltration may also occur. The disease may be idiopathic or may occur at sites of existing lesions.

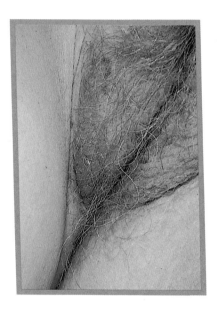

↑ **495 Amyloidosis** of vulva.

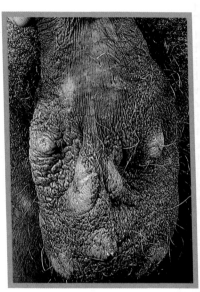

↑ **496 Leprosy of scrotum** cf. scrotal folliculitis (**465**).

Leprosy (Hansen's disease)

The cause of this chronic infectious condition is *Mycobacterium leprae* (Hansen's bacillus). Genital lesions are rare, but typical macules, papules, plaques and nodules may occur. The lesions are usually multiple and may be hypopigmented or slightly erythematous: anaesthesia is unusual. Usually other manifestations of leprosy are present.

INTERACTION BETWEEN HIV AND OTHER SEXUALLY TRANSMITTED DISEASES

The interactions between sexually transmitted diseases and HIV warrant special mention. They include: increased risk of transmission of HIV and other sexually transmitted diseases; altered clinical manifestations of sexually transmitted diseases in association with immunosuppression; and, possibly, more rapid progression of HIV disease itself due to sexually transmitted disease cofactors (**497**).

TRANSMISSION

It is clear that, worldwide, the predominant mode of transmission of HIV is by sexual activity (**498**). Furthermore, over the past decade, there has been increasing evidence that HIV transmission and acquisition can be facilitated by other sexually transmitted infections. Most epidemiological studies worldwide have indicated that the risk of acquiring HIV in the presence of concurrent sexually transmitted disease is increased by 2–6-fold. The risk has generally been higher with genital ulcer disease than with non-ulcerative sexually transmitted diseases, although the latter still cause a significant increase in relative risk in studies that have been carefully controlled for other factors, such as sexual behaviour and condom use.

The mechanisms explaining increased transmission are not yet fully understood, but there are at least two biologically plausible explanations. Firstly, HIV-positive men and women may have increased infectiousness due to an increased shedding of HIV from inflammatory and exudative sexually transmitted disease lesions. Secondly, one might expect an increased susceptibility of HIV-negative men and women to HIV because of the changes in the epithelial barriers of HIV target cells, such as T lymphocytes and macrophages, in conditions such as ulceration, micro-ulceration, cervical erosion and increased cervical friability (**499**).

CLINICAL EFFECTS

Clinical manifestations of many non-sexually transmitted diseases are often significantly altered in HIV disease, particularly as individuals become progressively more immunosuppressed (see p. 283). Not surprisingly, this can also happen with sexually transmitted infections in HIV-positive individuals. Clearly, more florid lesions or delayed healing (perhaps associated with an increased resistance to therapy) might be important in increasing the transmission of HIV. For example, chancroid is the predominant ulcerative condition in many countries in the developing world, and there is some evidence for larger, more persistent lesions and failure of some previously standard therapies in the presence of concurrent HIV disease. Alterations in natural history are of course important in their own right even if they do not facilitate HIV transmission. Examples include the rapid progression of cervical dysplasia

251

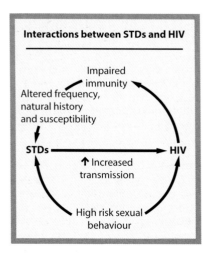

Interactions between STDs and HIV

← **497 Interactions between STDs and HIV.**

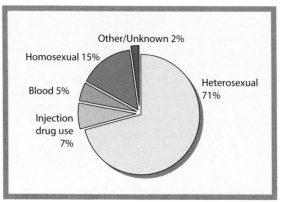

← **498 Proportion of cumulative adult HIV infections by mode of transmission**
Redrawn with permission from: Mann J, Tarantola DJM, Netter TW, (eds) *AIDS in the World*, Harvard University Press, Cambridge (Mass.) 1992

in patients with HIV co-infection; or more severe pelvic inflammatory disease (PID) in HIV disease as has been reported. Further examples are given later.

INTERVENTION
Several studies have been initiated in different countries to see whether increased facilities for the diagnosis and treatment of sexually transmitted infections will reduce some of the factors discussed above and so lower the incidence of HIV infection. The first study to be reported was from the Mwanza

region, Tanzania, with the results providing strong support for this hypothesis. The annual incidence of HIV was almost halved in this population from 1.9–1.2% per year. This 42% reduction was achieved with no appreciable change in condom usage which remained extremely low. However, other studies have shown that condom usage is effective in preventing HIV transmission. For example, sexually transmitted diseases, including HIV, were reduced by condom usage in a prostitute population in Zaire. Another study in Europe showed that HIV transmission could be prevented by consistent use of condoms in heterosexual couples of whom one partner was HIV positive.

CLINICAL EXAMPLES
Herpes simplex virus (HSV)
The recurrence of HSV infections becomes more frequent as HIV-positive patients become more immunosuppressed. Furthermore, virus isolates resistant to standard therapies, e.g. aciclovir, are found almost only in immunodeficient individuals. An example (**500**) is given of a patient, presenting in late 1986, who had intractable vulval and perianal herpes despite

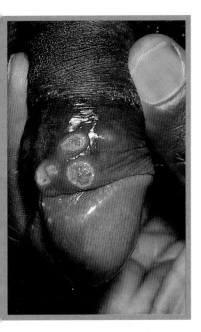

← 499 Chancroid
It is not surprising that ulcerative conditions, such as chancroid, are associated with an increased risk of transmission and acquisition of human immunodeficiency virus (HIV). There is also an increased risk associated with non-ulcerative STDs.

aciclovir therapy. Her herpes was shown to be caused by a thymidine kinase-negative mutant of HSV. Subsequently, she was given an antiretroviral drug (zidovudine), which produced a modest improvement in her immunity, as evidenced by an increase in her CD4-positive lymphocyte count. Although zidovudine has no antiherpetic effect, her herpetic lesions completely healed, confirming the effect of immunity on herpes simplex expression (**501**).

Other altered presentations of HSV infection include **disseminated herpes simplex**, which in our experience may lead to delayed diagnosis (**502, 503**). This illustrates a general point that, where feasible, biopsies should be performed for unusual HIV-associated skin lesions.

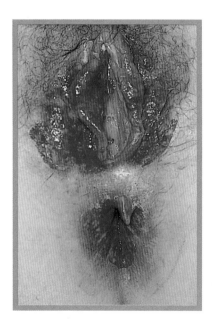

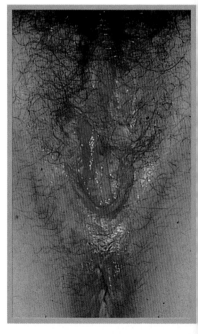

↑ 500 Severe vulval and perianal herpes in a patient with AIDS
The virus isolate was a thymidine kinase-negative mutant of herpes simplex and totally resistant to aciclovir.

↑ 501 Temporary resolution of herpetic lesions
seen in **500** following antiretroviral therapy (see text above).

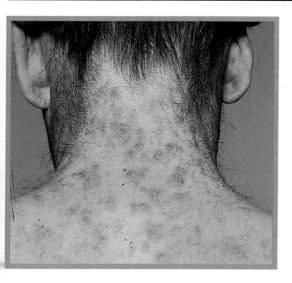

← 502
Generalized skin rash due to disseminated herpes simplex infection
HSV was confirmed by culture and biopsy. The patient's CD4-positive lymphocyte count was <100/mm^3 and the lesions responded well to aciclovir therapy.

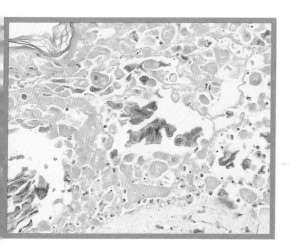

← 503
Histopathology of disseminated HSV lesions
High-power view of epidermis adjacent to an ulcer. The acanthocytes show the classical appearances of HSV infection with numerous moulded epidermal cells grouped together with ground-glass cytoplasm.

Molluscum contagiosum

Other chronic viral infections, such as molluscum contagiosum, may be extremely widespread and cosmetically distressing, particularly when they occur on the face (**504, 505**). They are often refractory to treatment.

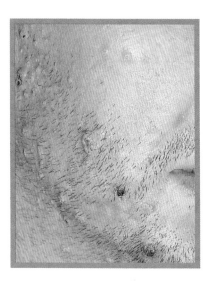

← 504 Severe molluscum contagiosum lesions
on the face in a patient with undetectable CD4-positive lymphocytes in the blood. Refractory to treatment.

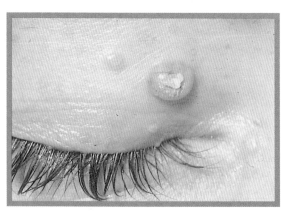

← 505 Giant molluscum contagiosum lesions
are not uncommon in HIV disease.

Papillomaviruses

These may also be more florid and difficult to eradicate. This relates to both genital warts (**506**) and non-genital warts. Papillomaviruses may also have carcinogenic potential. As well as **cervical dysplasia**, we have seen several cases of **squamous cell cloacogenic carcinoma of the anus (507)**.

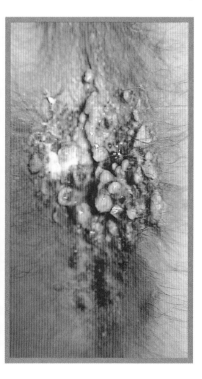

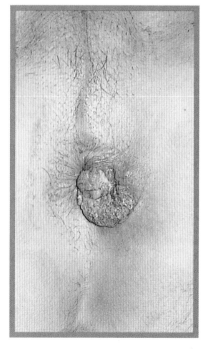

↑ **506 Florid genital wart virus infection**
in an immunocompromised patient.

↑ **507 Cloacogenic cell carcinoma (associated with human papillomavirus infection)**
in a patient with AIDS.

Syphilis

It is not yet clear how commonly, despite treatment, changes occur in the natural history of syphilis in terms of altered clinical expression, failure of early treatment or reactivation. However, there have been some anecdotal reports suggesting changes in clinical patterns. These include exuberant early lesions such as **punched-out (malignant) secondary syphilis** in an HIV-positive patient, reminiscent of the descriptions of early syphilis when it first appeared in Europe in the 16th century (**508, 509**). The patient responded well to standard penicillin therapy. We have also seen several patients with **tertiary syphilis** with a history of apparently adequate penicillin therapy for early disease many years previously. An example of a patient with **gummatous syphilis** is shown in **510**.

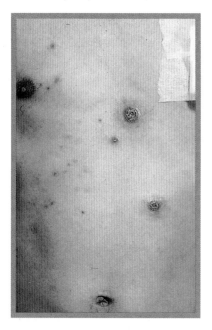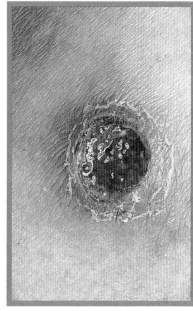

↑ **508, 509 Punched-out lesions of secondary syphilis**
in a South American patient. The patient was found to be coinfected with HIV.

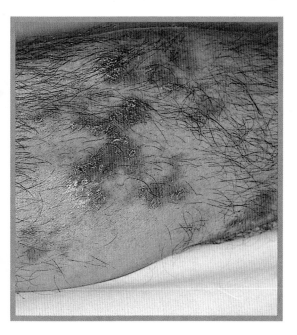

← **510**
Gummatous skin lesions (tertiary syphilis)
in a patient who gave a history of apparently adequate treatment for early syphilis some 20 years previously. This manifestation therefore could have been due to reactivation associated with increasing immunodeficiency. Alternatively, the patient could have been reinfected with syphilis at a subsequent date.

Ectoparasites

Finally, the response to ectoparasites may be markedly different in severely immunocompromised HIV-positive individuals due to skin anergy. The condition of **crusted scabies** is not uncommon but may not be immediately recognised. This is particularly important as crusted scabies is highly infectious

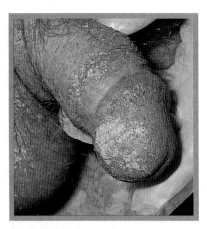
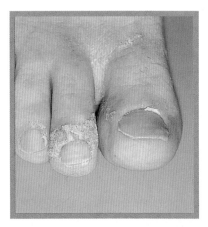
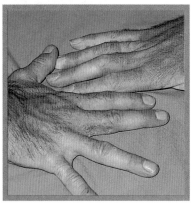
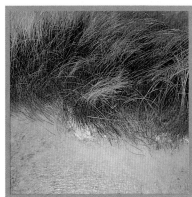

↑ 511–514 Examples of crusted scabies

These lesions are highly infectious. The scaly scalp was initially thought to be due to severe tinea capitis but was found to be teeming with mites.

to contacts, including medical and nursing attendants. This is due to the presence of millions of mites, as evidenced by the relative ease of finding mites on histological section. In biopsies from non-crusted scabies, mites are much more difficult to find (**511–515**).

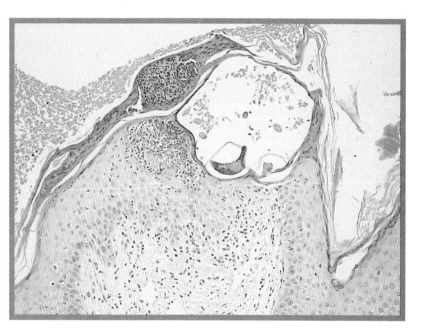

↑ 515 Scabetic mites
Histological section showing easily detected scabetic mites in a case of crusted scabies.

HUMAN IMMUNODEFICIENCY VIRUS (HIV) DISEASE

INTRODUCTION

We are now well into the second decade of the HIV/AIDS pandemic. Clinical recognition of the disease was first made in the USA in 1981 when the Centers for Disease Control (CDC), Atlanta, noticed increased requests for pentamidine to be used in the treatment of *Pneumocystis carinii* pneumonia (PCP) in young men. This had previously been a rare infection. From both the West and East coasts of the United States, cases were reported of both PCP and Kaposi's sarcoma (KS) in homosexual men, and soon after of PCP in injecting drug users of both sexes. At about the same time, similar cases of opportunistic infections and tumours began to be noted in Africans attending European centres for treatment. Further epidemiological investigations confirmed a major epidemic in Africa, with transmission being predominantly heterosexual. Retrospective investigations have since shown that the infection was present for some years before it was clinically recognized; the earliest example of this is the finding of HIV antibodies in a 1959 specimen of stored serum from Zaire.

Data from the World Health Organization (WHO) reported by mid-1996 (**516**) show that a similar proportion (just over one-third of cases) are reported from the African Continent and the USA. Europe and the rest of the Americas

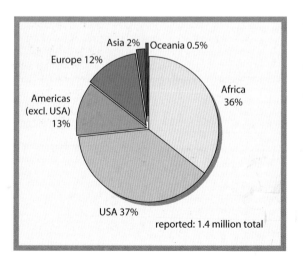

**← 516
Cumulative number of AIDS cases reported** in adults and children from the late 1970s to mid-1996. WHO data.

make up the bulk of the other cases. However, this picture changes dramatically if we look at the number of estimated cases of acquired immune deficiency syndrome (AIDS) (**517**). The predominance of the problem within Africa becomes only too apparent, making up almost three-quarters of the estimated disease burden. In Africa, AIDS is behaving like a sexually transmitted disease (**518**), with the highest rates occurring in early adult life and in urban as opposed to rural settings, and with the mean age of infected women being lower than that of men.

Worldwide, the epidemiological patterns are complex. Europe, like North America, has had a predominant involvement of homosexual men and injecting drug users, the latter generally outnumbering the former by 3 or 4:1 in southern Europe, the inverse being true for northern Europe. Extensive heterosexual transmission is well-established in South America and there are emerging epidemics of enormous significance in India, Thailand and other Asian countries.

It was a surprise to many observers that HIV took so long to become prevalent in Asia. However, this was not due to lack of effective documentation. For example, in Thailand, repeated serosurveillance studies showed little evidence of infection even in high-risk populations, such as injecting drug users. Then, in 1988, there was an explosive increase in prevalence from under 1% to 44% in less than a year (**519**). This was

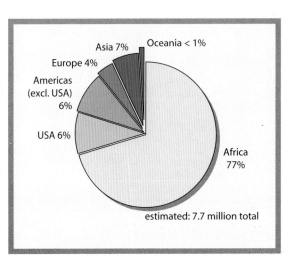

← 517
Cumulative number of AIDS cases estimated in adults and children from the late 1970s to mid-1996. WHO data.

followed by a parallel epidemic with a different clade (subtype) virus with successive waves of transmission in female prostitutes, their predominantly non-injecting drug user male clients and, within 1–2 years, the general heterosexual population. Subsequent careful epidemiological investigation in Changmai, north Thailand, confirmed a rapidly increasing prevalence in military recruits, although in latter years prevention efforts, including the '100% condom policy' have had remarkable success.

Transmission via blood products has been dramatically curtailed in many countries with the advent of universal HIV testing and asking patients to defer from giving blood if they feel they might be at any risk. However, in some countries, particularly those with professionally paid donors, there has been distressing evidence of continued transmission. Furthermore, in some areas, the reuse of contaminated medical equipment has been a significant source of new infections.

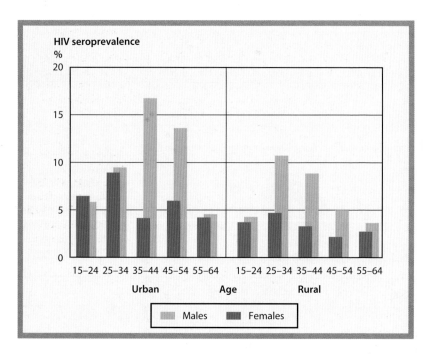

↑ 518 Epidemiology of HIV in Sierra Leone
Redrawn with permission from Mann J, (ed) *op. cit.*

Vertical transmission has been reported to occur in 13–37% of pregnancies in various studies, without antiretroviral intervention. In addition, many uninfected children will therefore become orphans , particularly in the developing world, over the next few years (**520**).

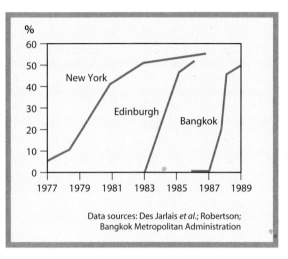

Data sources: Des Jarlais *et al.*; Robertson; Bangkok Metropolitan Administration

← 519 The rapid rise of HIV prevalence in injecting drug users in Bangkok in 1987–1988 was similar to previous epidemics in Europe and the USA. Subsequently, similar patterns occurred in other Asian countries. Redrawn with permission from GV Stimson.

25–30 million cumulative adult HIV infection
8–10 million cumulative adult AIDS cases

Plus
5–10 million cumulative paediatric HIV infections
4–8 million cumulative paediatric AIDS cases

Total
30–40 million cumulative HIV infections
in men, women and children

12–18 million cumulative AIDS cases
in men, women and children

In addition
10–15 million children younger than 15 years of age
may be orphaned as a result of maternal AIDS

← 520 Cumulative estimates for the year 2000—adults and children: WHO global programme on AIDS.

CAUSE

Previously known as lymphadenopathy-associated virus (LAV) and human T cell lymphotrophic virus III (HTLV III), the virus was isolated first in France (1983) and reported in the United States (1984). It is called a retrovirus because of the presence of the enzyme, reverse transcriptase. This enzyme converts the viral RNA to DNA, which then becomes integrated into the genome of the host cells. Human immunodeficiency virus type 1 (HIV 1) is the major cause of HIV disease throughout the world. A second virus, human immunodeficiency virus type 2 (HIV 2) was identified in 1985 in West African patients and a number of cases have now been reported in Europe, South America, India and North America. Interestingly, HIV 1 has only about 40% homology of nucleoside sequences with HIV 2 and is, in fact, more closely related genetically to the simian immune deficiency virus which occurs in chimpanzees (SIV_{CPZ}). HIV 2 is more closely related to the virus found in sooty mangabeys (SIV_{SMM}). Recently, a further human isolate, HIV 0, has been described from the Cameroon. This appears to be a variant of HIV 1 (**521–523**).

HIV subtypes

To date, nine HIV-1 subtypes have been identified, several with distinct geographical distributions: for example, subtypes A, C and D dominate in subSaharan Africa; E dominates in Thailand; and B in the USA and Western Europe. There is laboratory evidence that the African and Asian subtypes may be biologically particularly well-adapted to sexual transmission, which may be an additional factor contributing to the extent of the heterosexual epidemics in these continents.

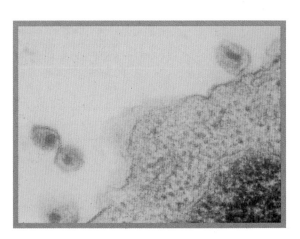

← 521 Mature virions of HIV seen budding from an infected lymphocyte in cell culture.

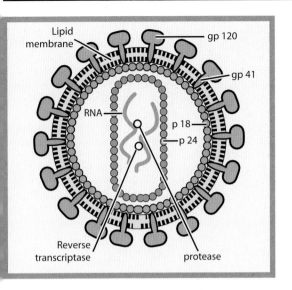

← **522 Drawing of HIV showing main components.**

Lipid membrane
gp 120
gp 41
RNA
p 18
p 24
Reverse transcriptase
protease

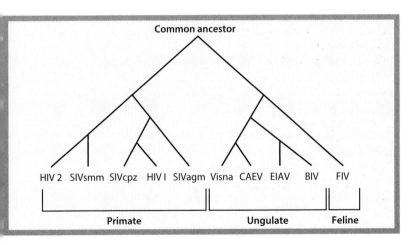

Common ancestor

HIV 2 SIVsmm SIVcpz HIV I SIVagm Visna CAEV EIAV BIV FIV

Primate   Ungulate   Feline

↑ **523 Phylogenetic tree**
showing approximate relationship between some cytopathic retroviruses (lentiviruses). See page 266: SIV=simian immunodeficiency virus; SMM=sooty mangabey; CPZ=chimpanzee; AGM=african green monkey.

TRANSMISSION OF INFECTION

HIV has been recovered from most body fluids (blood, semen, vaginal fluid, lymphocytes, saliva, urine, tears, breast milk, cerebrospinal fluid, synovial fluid, plasma). However, the concentration of virus (probably related to infectivity) is very variable. There is evidence that the viral load is greatest at the time of seroconversion and then again during the later stages of disease (**524**), and transmission by whatever route may be greater at these times.

In practice, transmission has only occurred through the following methods: penetrative sexual contact; via blood products administered by transfusion (before the introduction of screening for HIV antibodies); in needle-sharing (injecting drug users and therapeutic use); from mother to child *in utero* and at delivery (with a modest additional risk from breast feeding).

HIV 1 and HIV 2 are cytopathic viruses, although the latter appears to be less pathogenic with a more slowly evolving clinical course. HIV 2 is also less readily transmitted by whatever mode of transmission. Coinfection is possible although recent evidence suggests natural infection with HIV 2 confers some protection against HIV 1 superinfection

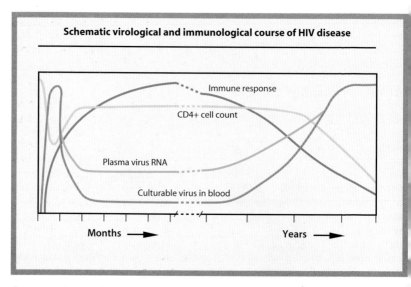

↑ 524 Schematic virological and immunological course of HIV disease redrawn with permission from: Saag MS et al., HIV vital load markers in clinical practice. *Nature* (Commentary and Review); **2**;6;p.625

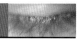

IMMUNOLOGY

It was noted soon after the discovery of HIV that it specifically attaches to cells bearing CD4 receptors on their surface. These cells include, in particular, T helper lymphocytes (CD4 cells), monocyte/macrophages, and their counterparts within the central nervous system. The virus is thus lymphotrophic and neurotrophic. The mechanism of infection is still not completely understood, although a number of additional receptors, including the chemokine receptors CXCR4 (fusin) and CCR5 have now been described (see also p. 269). Initial infection by macrophage trophic (also called non-syncytium-inducing or NSI) HIV strains appear to require the CCR5 chemokine receptor. Then, at a later stage, HIV switches its trophism from macrophages and T-cells to T-cells alone (also called syncytium-inducing or SI) HIV strains, which utilise the CXCR4 receptor.

In the sexual context, there are numerous susceptible cells within the genital and/or rectal mucosa. The number of these susceptible cells are augmented in the presence of coexistent sexually transmitted diseases (see p. 269). Infected cells are then likely to migrate to lymph nodes leading to a chronic, persistent infection, progressive immune deficiency and AIDS. Clearly, much of the immune defect in late-stage disease can be attributed to low absolute numbers of CD4-positive T lymphocytes. In addition, there are qualitative changes in CD4-positive T cell function, also reducing cell-mediated immunity. This results in an increased susceptibility to tumours and infections, particularly fungal and viral diseases, prevalent in HIV disease,

SEROLOGICAL DIAGNOSIS

Several screening tests, e.g. enzyme immunoassays (EIA), particle agglutination assays (PIA), have been developed to detect one or more of the antibodies (usually antiHIV envelope (gp120) IgG) produced in HIV infection: many are relatively simple technically. Fortunately, results are both sensitive and specific and, therefore, are likely to remain reliable even in populations with a low prevalence of HIV infection. Later-generation tests are somewhat more sensitive and a positive antiHIV may develop within 3–4 weeks after infection but, more commonly, it appears at about 6 weeks. It may, however, be delayed for up to 6 months and very occasionally may take longer to appear. During pre-test discussion, it is important that patients realize that the antiHIV test produces a variable response. In practice, when the history suggests a low risk of HIV infection, the authors feel that a negative test at 3 months is usually adequate. However, with a higher risk exposure, or other factors, then the test should probably be repeated at least at 6 months.

Given the significance of a positive test, we feel it is important to test specimens found positive on screening with at least one other different method; if both these tests give positive results, a further specimen, taken on a separate occasion, should be retested by the same methods. Testing should only be undertaken after pre-test advice to ensure that patients fully understand the implication of the test result: post-test counselling will often also be necessary.

Currently used tests cover all known HIV viruses, including HIV 1, HIV 2, and the recently described HIV 0 (a subtype of HIV 1) from the Cameroon. It will be important to maintain vigilance as new HIV variants are described. In cases of suspected seroconversion illness, antigen detection tests should be used as they become positive prior to the development of antibodies. These include an EIA for HIV p24 core antigen and the HIV viral load assays, e.g. HIV RNA genome polymerase chain reaction.

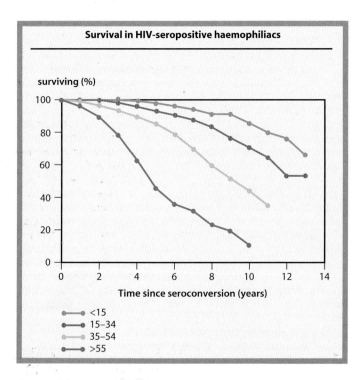

↑ **525 Survival in HIV-seropositive haemophilia patients by age at seroconversion** From: Darby et al. Importance of age at infection with HIV 1 for survival and development of AIDS in UK haemophiliac population. Lancet, 1996;**347**;1573–1579.

NATURAL HISTORY OF HIV INFECTION

The average length of time from HIV infection to development of AIDS in developed countries is about 10 years, with no major differences between various transmission groups. However, there is a strong association with age in that older individuals tend to progress more quickly. In a recent study in haemophiliacs, survival at 10 years among patients who seroconverted at ages under 15 years, 15–34 years, 35–54 years, and over 55 years was 86%, 72%, 45% and 12%, respectively (**525**). In addition, a subgroup of neonates who had probably acquired the infection *in utero* rather than perinatally have a shortened time course. There are also geographical differences that partly depend on the different prevalence of conventional and opportunistic infections, but perhaps more importantly, lack of access to medical care and expensive drugs. Thus, in Africa and other developing countries, a significantly higher morbidity is expected in early HIV disease with a predominance of prevalent high-grade pathogens (those that are sufficiently virulent to cause disease in immunocompetent individuals). These include infections, such as *Mycobacterium tuberculosis, Streptococcus pneumoniae*, shigella and salmonella which may lead to an early death due to the lack of ready diagnosis and treatment.

There is considerable variation in time in the rate of progression to symptomatic disease. Some investigators have postulated cofactors, such as coexisting infective agents, but none has been proven. Genetic cofactors may be important and individuals with certain major histocompatibility antigens appear to be relatively protected. Genetic variation in the chemokine receptor CCR5 sheds some light on both infection and progression in certain individuals. Thus homozygous deletion of part of the CCR5 gene appears to account for resistance to HIV infection for some multiply-exposed people. In addition, heterozygotes with reduced CCR5 expression may have delayed progression to disease. Currently, there is much research into the so-called 'non-progressors' who persist with high levels of CD4-positive T cells, but it is not known yet whether these individuals are just at the extreme of the normal distribution curve for development of HIV-related disease and AIDS.

DEFINITIONS/CLASSIFICATION

A number of case definitions of AIDS and classification systems for HIV infection have been developed. These include the Centers for Disease Control (CDC) classification, which has been accepted by the WHO (**526**).

For surveillance purposes, a number of conditions were defined as AIDS indicator diseases; these have been augmented over the years. The CDC also suggested that individuals with CD4 counts under 200/mm^3 should also be defined as having AIDS. Clearly, funding and access for these tests may not be available in many parts of the world. To accommodate local circumstances, the WHO has developed a number of clinical case definitions, as well as its own clinical/laboratory staging system for HIV infection.

Prognostic laboratory markers

Quantitative measurements of viral load by a number of different techniques currently give the best predicted values for disease progression, while changes in viral load are best for predicting therapeutic response. This is particularly true at higher levels of CD4 count when the latter is a poor predictor of prognosis. However, the CD4 lymphocyte count (absolute or percentage) at lower counts is useful both prognostically and in deciding when to begin primary prophylaxis against several opportunistic infections.

**CDC/WHO classification system for HIV infection
and disease in adolescents and adults**

	Clinical Categories		
CD4+ T-cell categories	(A) Asymptomatic or PGL	(B) Symptomatic, not (A) or (C) conditions	(C) AIDS-indicator conditions
1 ≥ 500/mm³	A1	B1	C1
2 200-499/mm³	A2	B2	C2
3 < 200/mm³	A3	B3	C3

NB Categories are defined by both CD4 count and clinical presentation.
Shaded area indicates AIDS
Where there is an overlap of conditions, (C) takes precedence over (B),
which takes precedence over (A).
For classification purposes, once a category B condition has occurred, the
subject will remain in category B. The same goes for progression to
category C.

Category A
- Asymptomatic HIV infection
- Persistent generalised lymphadenopathy
- Acute (primary) HIV infection with accompanying illness or history of
  acute HIV infection

Category B
- Bacillary angiomatosis
- Candidiasis, oropharyngeal (thrush)
- Candidiasis, vulvovaginal; persistent, frequent or poorly responsive to
  therapy
- Cervical dysplasia (moderate or severe)/cervical carcinoma *in situ*
- Constitutional symptoms, such as fever (38.5 °C) or diarrhoea lasting >1
  month
- Hairy leukoplakia, oral
- Herpes zoster (shingles), involving at least two distinct episodes of more
  than one dermatome
- Idiopathic thrombocytopenic purpura
- Listeriosis
- Pelvic inflammatory disease, particularly if complicated by tubo-ovarian
  abscess
- Peripheral neuropathy

↑ **526 Current CDC classifications of HIV, 1993 (contd. overleaf).**

Category C

- Candidiasis of bronchi, trachea or lungs
- Candidiasis, oesophageal
- Cervical cancer, invasive
- Coccidioidomycosis, disseminated or extrapulmonary
- Cryptococcosis, extrapulmonary
- Cytomegalovirus disease (other than liver, spleen or nodes)
- Cytomegalovirus retinitis (with loss of vision)
- Encephalopathy, HIV-related
- Herpes simplex: chronic ulcer(s) (>1 month duration); or bronchitis, pneumonitis or oesophagitis
- Histoplasmosis, disseminated or extrapulmonary
- Isosporiasis, chronic intestinal (>1 month duration)
- Kaposi's sarcoma
- Lymphoma, Burkitt (or equivalent term)
- Lymphoma, immunoblastic (or equivalent term)
- Lymphoma, primary, of brain
- *Mycobacterium avium* complex or *M. kansasii*, disseminated or extrapulmonary
- *Mycobacterium tuberculosis*, any site (pulmonary or extrapulmonary)
- *Mycobacterium*, other species or unidentified species, disseminated or extrapulmonary
- *Pneumocystitis carinii* pneumonia
- Pneumonia, recurrent
- Progressive multifocal leukoencephalopathy
- *Salmonella* septicaemia, recurrent
- Toxoplasmosis of brain
- Wasting syndrome due to HIV

↑ **526 Current CDC classifications of HIV, 1993 (contd.).**

PRIMARY HIV INFECTION (CDC CATEGORY A)

There is increasing recognition that symptomatic seroconversion is the rule rather than the exception, although it is often not recognized and dismissed as a trivial 'viral infection'. It is now known that there is a period of intense viral replication before the onset of immune response and clinical illness, which may develop 1–4 weeks after exposure to HIV. At this stage, patients will usually have a positive p24 antigen and negative antibody tests with perhaps evolving bands on the Western blot. Patients may present with general features, including **fever**, **night sweats** and **myalgia**, but also with **specific involvement of the skin, gut and nervous system**. **Lethargy** and **malaise** are frequent and in a recent treatment study of patients presenting with HIV seroconversion illness, the mean length of symptoms was 1 month with some patients having had symptoms for several months. The clinical features of primary HIV infection are shown in the table (**527**) and the figure (**528**).

General	Dermatologic
Fever	Erythematous maculopapular rash (symmetrical, usually affects face/trunk also palms/soles)
Pharyngitis	
Lymphadenopathy	
Arthralgia	Roseola-like rash
Myalgia	Diffuse urticaria
Lethargy/malaise	Desquamation
Anorexia/weight loss	Alopecia
	Mucocutaneous ulceration

Gastrointestinal	Neuropathic
Oral candida	Headache/ retro-orbital pain
Nausea/vomiting	
Diarrhoea	Aseptic meningitis/ encephalitis
Hepatitis	Peripheral neuropathy
	Radiculopathy
	Guillain-Barré syndrome
	Cognitive/ affective impairments

← **527 Summary of general, gastrointestinal, neuropathic and dermatological manifestations of HIV.**

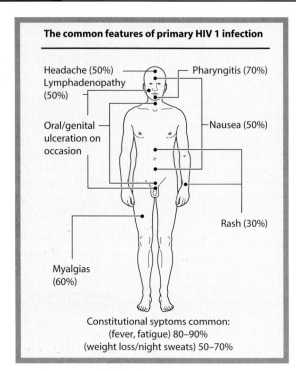

The common features of primary HIV 1 infection

Headache (50%)
Lymphadenopathy (50%)
Pharyngitis (70%)
Oral/genital ulceration on occasion
Nausea (50%)
Rash (30%)
Myalgias (60%)

Constitutional syptoms common:
(fever, fatigue) 80–90%
(weight loss/night sweats) 50–70%

← 528 The features of primary HIV 1 infection.

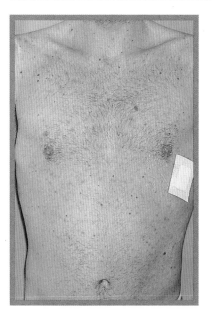

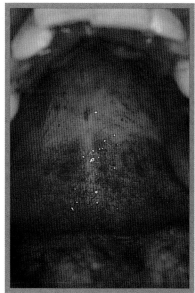

↑ 529, 530 Primary HIV 1 infection
These photographs show the same patient, who presented with a widespread maculopapular rash with prominent involvement of the palms of his hands. The differential diagnosis therefore included secondary syphilis and other viral exanthemata. Initially HIV antibody tests were negative; HIV p24 antigen was equivocal but this became definitely positive 1 week later (see **524**).

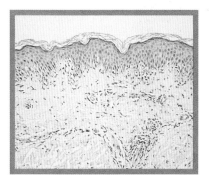

← 531 Skin biopsy from the same patient as shown in 529 and 530
Epidermis showing an interface dermatitis with basal spongiosis and cell apoptosis with an associated mild perivascular chronic inflammatory infiltrate. The appearances are of a viral exanthema although a drug-related rash could produce similar histological features.

Asymptomatic infection with or without persistent generalized lymphadenopathy (PGL) (CDC Category A)

After the viraemia associated with primary HIV infection, there usually follows a period of **clinical latency** when patients are relatively asymptomatic. It is a period of marked immune activation and control of HIV, mostly within the lymph nodes. Clinically, a substantial proportion of patients will have **PGL**, which is defined as an enlargement (more than 1 cm) of lymph nodes in at least two extrainguinal sites persisting for more than 3 months (**532**). At one time, this was thought to have prognostic significance, but prospective studies have shown that asymptomatic HIV-positive patients, with and without PGL , progress to AIDS at a similar rate. The enlarged glands are usually discrete, firm and may ache or be slightly tender. At times, they are a cause of initial presentation or they may only be detected after careful clinical examination; the most common sites are cervical, postauricular and axillary, but any site may be involved including epitrochlear nodes. A CT scan of the abdomen may show enlargement of the retroperitoneal glands. It is important to remember that there are many causes for lymphadenopathy; investigation of suspect cases must be comprehensive.

Some patients with PGL remain relatively well for years; glandular enlargement may fluctuate in size but there is no significant change in general

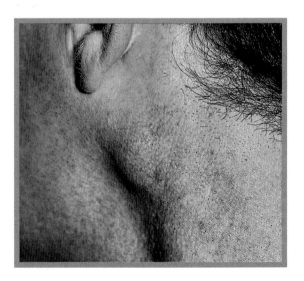

← **532 Persistent generalized lymphadenopathy (PGL).**

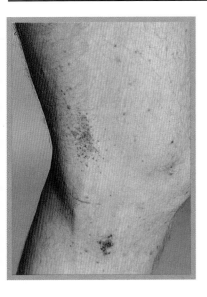

← 533 Thrombocytopenia purpura
Asymptomatic thrombocytopenia between 50 000–150 000 is common. At times, counts drop lower to become clinically significant and purpuric lesions may also develop.

health. In other patients, there are symptoms (fatiguability, fever, diarrhoea) which may progress to more overt symptomatic disease. Immunologically and prognostically, there is considerable overlap between asymptomatic and symptomatic disease. Specific laboratory investigations such as CD4-positive lymphocyte counts and HIV viral load aid prognosis.

Routine laboratory investigation may show minor haematological changes, such as a modest degree of **lymphopenia** or **thrombocytopenia** (**533**). Biopsy of enlarged glands is generally unhelpful, showing non-specific follicular hyperplasia unless specific stains are performed (**534**). However, gland biopsy is useful to exclude other causes of lymphadenopathy, particularly with enlarging or fixed glands or to investigate coexistent hilar lymphadenopathy.

Symptomatic disease
As HIV disease progresses, there is a gradual decrease in immune function, particularly a drop in CD4-positive lymphocyte count. Patients are constitutionally unwell with intermittent or more persistent complications which were previously called **AIDS-related complex** (**ARC**). Both clinical and laboratory markers need to be taken into consideration when defining someone's prognosis. The distinction between symptomatic non-AIDS disease and AIDS is blurred and there is much overlap between the clinical stages, which may become more marked with more extensive use of primary prophylaxis against opportunistic infections (**535**).

Constitutional symptoms of HIV disease due to increasing cellular immune deficiency include: loss of body weight; night sweats; persistent pyrexia; persistent diarrhoea; herpes zoster, sometimes occurring simultaneously in two or three dermatomes; recrudescence of herpes simplex (especially perianal); a variety of dermatological problems; oral candidiasis; and the apparently unique oral lesion hairy leukoplakia (OHL), caused by reactivation of Epstein–Barr virus (EBV).

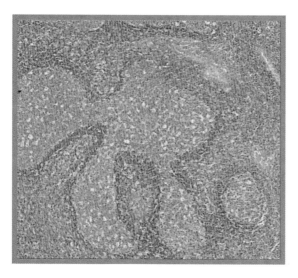

← 534 Persistent generalized lymphaden-opathy
Histopathology (medium power) of lymph node showing marked reactive hyperplasia and irregular germinal centre and encroachment of mantle zone lymphocytes into germinal centre (see **532**).

Acquired immune deficiency syndrome (AIDS)
(CDC, Categories A3 B3 C)

In advanced HIV disease, there is severe immune deficiency with increasing viraemia. As mentioned previously, a number of conditions have been determined for surveillance purposes to define AIDS (**526**). The clinical manifestations of AIDS will vary geographically depending on the prevalence of different infections in various parts of the world (**536**). In addition, the risk of developing an opportunistic infection also depends on the pathogenicity of the microorganism. Thus, *Mycobacterium tuberculosis* (MTB) infection may occur at any stage of HIV disease, whereas disseminated *Mycobacterium avium complex* (MAC) infection, **cytomegalovirus** (CMV) infection and **microsporidiosis** tend to only occur in patients with marked immunosuppression and CD4 counts less than $50/mm^3$. Opportunistic tumours, such as **non-Hodgkin's lymphoma**, are also more common at lower CD4 counts, but may occur earlier (**537**).

Survival after AIDS diagnosis, like the AIDS incubation period, is extremely variable: once again, older patients generally progress more rapidly. Other factors include specific AIDS diagnosis, treatment, and subsequent secondary prophylaxis of infections, but discussion of these is outside the scope of this book. There are currently rapid changes in the field of antiretroviral therapy (and immune-based treatments) against HIV, which may have dramatic effects on prognosis in those parts of the world able to institute and monitor such therapies.

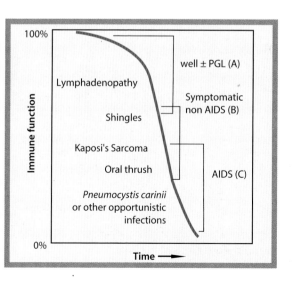

← 535 The decline of immune function with time
AIDS diagnoses vary depending on prevailing pathogens. Primary prophylaxis may delay their appearance.

The range of presentations of HIV disease is extremely wide and what follows in this book represents examples of presentations both common and rare, predominantly from the authors' UK experience.

Opportunistic infections and their incidence in different populations		
Infections	**Incidence**	
	High	**Low**
Tuberculosis	Injecting drug users Developing world Poor social conditions Prisons	Gay men BCG vaccinated
Pneumocystosis	Developed world No prophylaxis	Prophylaxis Developing world
Toxoplasmosis	Countries where raw meat is frequently consumed	
Cryptococcosis	Developing world	Europe
Other systemic mycoses	Endemic areas (USA, South America)	
Cryptosporidiosis Microsporidiosis	Endemic areas	
Cytomegalovirus infection	Gay men	Developing world
Non-tuberculous mycobacteriosis		Developing world

↑ **536 Manifestations of AIDS vary depending on the prevalence of microorganisms in different geographical regions**
Prior places of habitation and travel are important parts of the medical history.

CD4 positive lymphocyte counts: risk of developing opportunistic infections or tumours	
CD4 Count	Opportunistic infection/tumour
> 200 *	*Mycobacterium* tuberculosis
	Kaposi's sarcoma
	Cryptosporidia—will resolve
< 200*	Non Hodgkin's lymphoma
	Pneumocystis carinii
	Oesophageal candida
	Toxoplasma
	Cryptococcus
<50	Disseminated systemic mycosis
	Cytomegalovirus retinitis
	Disseminated non-tuberculous mycobacteria (MAC)
	Microsporidia

*All can clearly occur at lower CD4 counts. Cryptosporidia may then produce chronic diarrhoea.

← 537 CD4 positive lymphocyte counts: risk of developing opportunistic infections or tumours.

CLINICAL MANIFESTATIONS OF HIV DISEASE
Pulmonary disease
There is a wide spectrum of lung disorders in AIDS, with important geographical variations (**536**). The commonest opportunistic infection found is *Pneumocystis carinii* **pneumonia** (**PCP**), although the advent of widespread use of primary prophylaxis against PCP in many parts of the world, including North America and Europe, has decreased this condition as an initial presentation of AIDS to below 50% of all diagnoses (**538**). A typical presentation of a patient with PCP is often insidious with shortness of breath and a non-productive cough. A chest X-ray may be normal or show widespread infiltration associated with profound hypoxia. Specific diagnosis may be made by an induced sputum (**539**) and/or bronchoscopy with bronchiolar lavage or transbronchial biopsy (**540**).

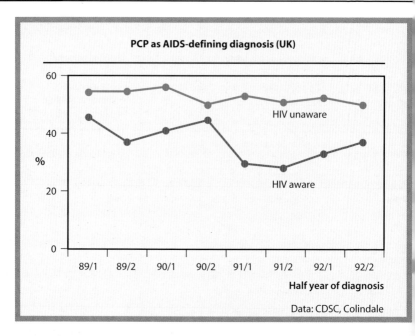

PCP as AIDS-defining diagnosis (UK)

HIV unaware

HIV aware

%

89/1 89/2 90/1 90/2 91/1 91/2 92/1 92/2

Half year of diagnosis

Data: CDSC, Colindale

↑ 538 *Pneumocystis carinii* **pneumonia (PCP)**
as initial AIDS-defining diagnosis (UK) in HIV-unaware and HIV-aware patients.
Reduction in PCP is mainly due to primary prophylaxis .

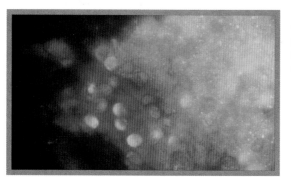

← **539 Induced
sputum specimen
showing *P. carinii***
demonstrated by
immunofluorescence.

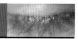

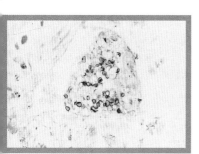

↑ **540 *P. carinii* in alveolus of lung biopsy**
stained with a silver stain.

↑ **541 Specific tests for tuberculosis (TB)**
should also be performed as a dual infection may occur. Here, a Ziehl–Nielsen stain of lung shows numerous acid-fast bacilli (morphology compatible with MTB and confirmed on culture).

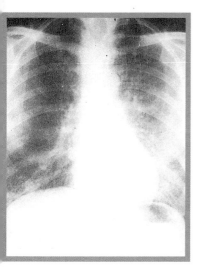

↑ **542 Chest X-ray of a patient with *P. carinii***
Bilateral ground-glass opacification which is more confluent in the left mid zone. Patient was hypoxic with a PO_2 <8 kPa.

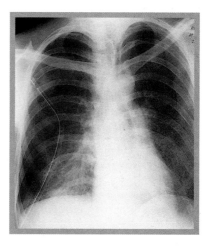

↑ **543 Pneumothorax**
is a common complication of *P. carinii*.

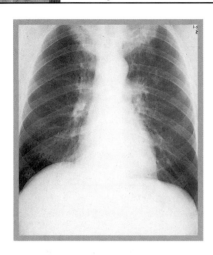

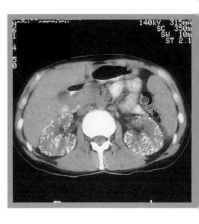

↑ **545** *P. carinii* **can disseminate widely**
Visceral involvement may lead to cystic lesions that appear calcified, as shown in the kidneys in this CT scan with multiple, bilateral lesions. Choroidal involvement may also be seen on ophthalmoscopy and may be confused with cottonwool spots (see **591**).

↑ **544 Upper lobe involvement with *P. carinii* masquerading as TB**
This may occur in the context of inhaled pentamidine being given as PCP prophylaxis, but which is not sufficiently protecting the upper lobes. There is also a risk of disseminated disease.

Other opportunistic infections include a wide range of: bacteria, such as *Mycobacterium tuberculosis* (MTB) and *Mycobacterium avium complex* (MAC), often with extrapulmonary lesions; protozoa, such as **Toxoplasma**; and fungi, such as **Aspergillus** and the various endemic mycoses, e.g. *Penicillium marneffei*, the latter often presenting as part of a disseminated disease. **Pneumonia** caused by traditional bacterial pathogens, such as the **pneumococci** are also considerably more common in HIV-positive individuals; these organisms may also cause sinusitis or occult bacteraemias (as has been described particularly in African patients).

It is estimated that several million people are coinfected with HIV and MTB. These individuals are at increased risk of both reactivation of latent infection and also accelerated progression of primary tuberculosis. Futhermore, marked immune activation with TB appears to increase HIV expression. Anergy may modify results of skin-testing.

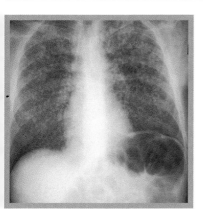

← 546 Miliary tuberculosis (TB) in an HIV-positive patient.

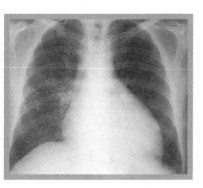

← 547 Globular heart shadow due to TB pericarditis
This is a common presentation of HIV in African and other endemic areas.

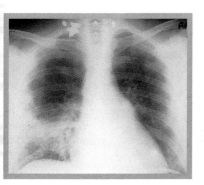

← 548 Richt middle lobe pneumococcal pneumonia
Chest X-ray shows right mid-zone shadowing obscuring the right heart border. This and other manifestations of pneumococcal infection are more common in HIV disease.

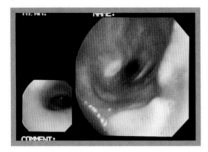

← 549 Aspergillus infection
appears to be not uncommon in late-stage HIV disease, not always associated with neutropenia or steroid therapy. Biopsy of these suggestive plaques seen on bronchoscopy confirmed the diagnosis.

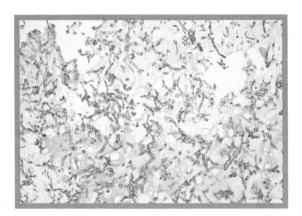

← 550 Aspergillus infection: fungal hyphae
showing characteristic 45° branching of septate hyphae with a PAS stain.

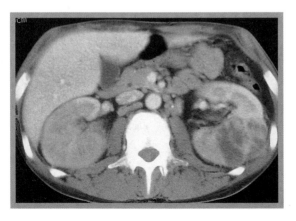

← 551 Disseminated Aspergillus
can occur, as with the kidney involvement shown in this CT scan. There is a large complex low-attenuation mass in the left kidney, with diffuse low attenuation and poor enhancement of the right kidney.

Non-infective lung disease includes **disseminated Kaposi's sarcoma** (which along with **TB** is the commonest cause of pleural effusions), **non-Hodgkin's lymphomas** and **lymphoid interstitial pneumonia** (more common in children than in adults).

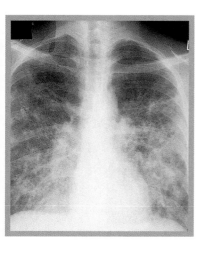

← 552 Kaposi's sarcoma involving the lung
Typical coarse infiltrates seen in the mid and lower zones.

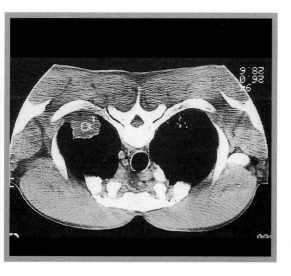

← 553 Non-Hodgkin's lymphoma: CT scan showing upper lobe mass lesion
The chest X-ray was suggestive of pulmonary TB but sputum culture was negative and the patient did not respond to empirical therapy. CT-guided biopsy of the lesions revealed non-Hodgkin's lymphoma.

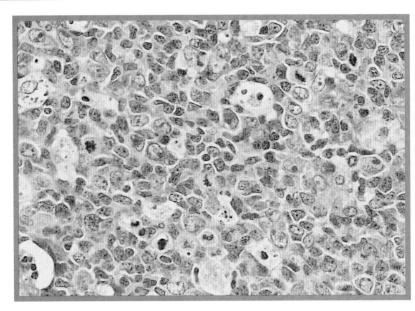

↑ 554 Histology of non-Hodgkin's lymphoma shown in 553
This high-power view shows a high-grade non-Hodgkin's lymphoma with many of the large cells showing prominent nucleoli.

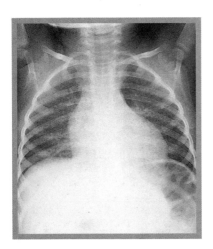

←555 Lymphoid interstitial pneumonitis
showing the characteristic multiple miliary opacities. This condition is more common in children.

MALIGNANT DISEASE
Kaposi's sarcoma (KS)

This condition has been recognised for many years as a multifocal, vascular tumour, initially described in elderly males with an East European Jewish ancestry as 'classic Kaposi's sarcoma'. The disease was relatively benign and affected mainly the skin of the lower extremities; patients usually died from other causes. Subsequently, KS was found to be endemic in subSaharan Africa, where the clinical manifestations were more varied and often followed a more aggressive course. Endemic disease was typically more severe in young children, with involvement of the lymphatic system and internal organs, and it has a much poorer prognosis. In the 1970s, occasional cases were described in patients immunosuppressed for renal transplantation, with the lesions often regressing when immunosuppressive therapy was removed. The link with immunosuppression was strengthened from 1981 onwards with the occurrence of increasing numbers of cases particularly in young men as the AIDS epidemic evolved.

In the United States, KS is at least 20 000 times more common in persons with AIDS than in the general population and 300 times more common than in other immunosuppressed groups. There was early epidemiological evidence that KS in AIDS might be caused by an interaction between HIV and a sexually transmitted cofactor, as KS was commoner among those who had acquired HIV via sexual contacts than parenterally, with a particularly high prevalence in homosexual and bisexual men. Women were more likely to have KS if their partners were bisexual men rather than injecting drug users. A few cases have also been described in HIV-negative homosexuals. Over the past few years, a candidate cofactor in the form of a new **herpes virus** (**KSHV**) has been been reported to have been found in the KS tissue of classical, endemic KS, as well as AIDS-associated KS. However, KSHV viral sequences have also been found in association with other tumours and the full aetiological significance has not yet been unravelled.

The most common **KS lesions** are easily visible, occurring in the **dermis** and the **oral cavity**. In many cases, there are also **systemic manifestations** in the **alimentary tract** or **lung**s which are often clinically silent initially. Lesions often begin as thickened dusky-red plaques which enlarge to raised nodules, often with a yellowish halo suggestive of old bruising. The lesions are usually painless, but may itch slightly: profuse bleeding can occur with trauma. Common sites include the lower limbs, the soles of the feet, the penis, the palate and the tip of the nose. In some cases, the lesions appear to be distributed along the lines of cleavage. The diagnosis is usually obvious on clinical grounds, but where possible a biopsy should be performed to confirm the diagnosis. KS may be the sole manifestation of AIDS at presentation and may occur when laboratory tests suggest a relatively preserved immune system (**535, 536**). More extensive lesions, visceral involvement and concurrent opportunistic infections are all associated with a worse prognosis.

Management of KS will depend on the extent of the disease. Infrequent skin lesions may be excised, treated with cryotherapy or intralesional or topical chemotherapy, with radiotherapy and systemic chemotherapy reserved for more widespread disease.

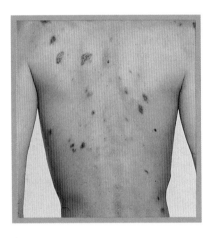

↑ 556 Kaposi's sarcoma (KS)
Early lesions. Note raised appearance.

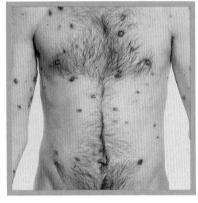

↑ 557 KS
Generalized lesions. Note peripheral bruising.

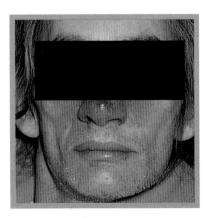

← 558 KS on tip of nose
Note also wasting, seborrhoeic dermatitis and angular cheilitis.

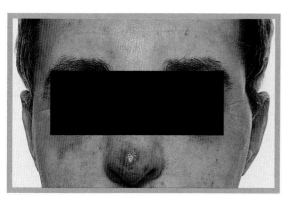

← 559 KS on tip of nose
Note also facial folliculitis.

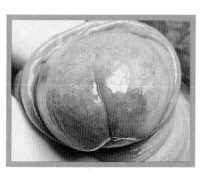

← 560 KS of glans penis, simulating balanitis (cf. **244**, **351**).

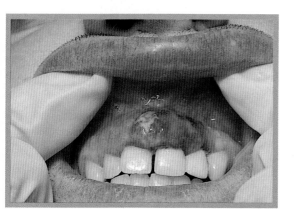

← 561 KS of gingivum.

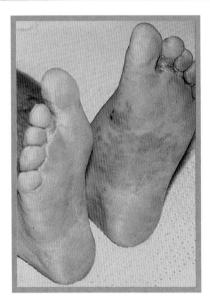

← 562 Kaposi's sarcoma (KS): discoloration of instep
Compare with secondary syphilis (see **106**).

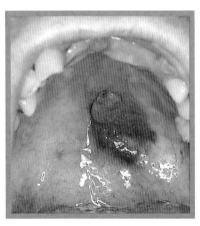

↑ 563 KS of palate
These lesions were clinically silent; the patient was referred by a dental surgeon, diagnosis '?AIDS'.

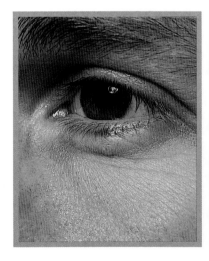

↑ 564 KS of lower eyelid
Subtle pigmented lesion.

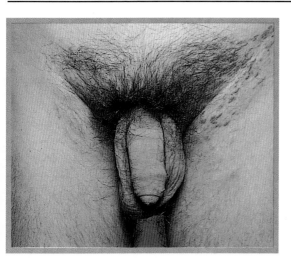

← 565 KS involving the lymph nodes in the groin

This may lead to blockage of the lymphatics and oedema of the genitalia and/or the lower limb. Radiotherapy to the groin may provide palliation.

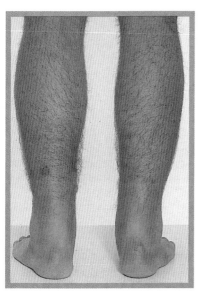

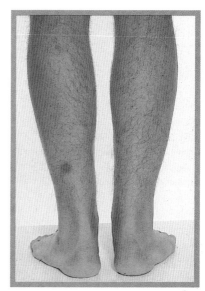

↑ 566, 567 KS showing lower limb oedema, before and after palliative radiotherapy to the groin.

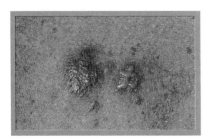

← 568 Kaposi's sarcoma (KS) lesions on the back

in close proximity to recurrent herpes simplex type 1.

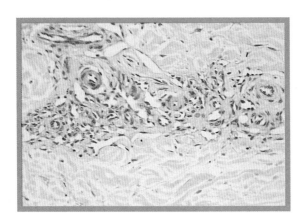

←569 Histopathology of KS

early lesion in the skin showing arborising irregular vessel dissecting collagen.

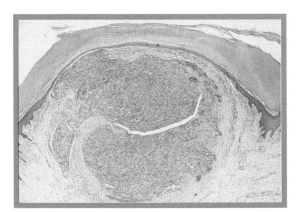

← 570 Histopathology of KS

low-power view of a classical type nodular KS.

Non-Hodgkin's lymphoma

Non-Hodgkin's lymphoma (NHL) is the second most common HIV-associated malignancy. Unlike KS, it can occur across all risk groups. In the developed world, it makes up 1–2% of all AIDS diagnoses and an increase in cases might be expected with prolonged survival at low levels of immunity. NHL in AIDS is a B lymphocyte neoplasm usually of unfavourable histological grade.

Central nervous system (CNS) NHL is usually a B lymphocyte neoplasm, associated with the Epstein–Barr virus, but this does not seem to be the case with all peripheral NHLs. CNS lymphomas often present late and are part of the differential diagnosis of CNS mass lesions (see p. 299). The prognosis is usually poor.

Peripheral NHL may occur in lymph nodes (which can enlarge with frightening speed), but in contrast to non-HIV infected patients, it is more likely to be extralymphatic, occurring in many sites, including the liver, rectum, duodenum, lung and mucocutaneous tissues. The symptoms depend on the site involved and diagnosis is usually established by biopsy. Although peripheral NHL can be seen at any stage of HIV disease, the median count in one series was approximately 200 CD4-positive lymphocytes per mm^3. Treatment will depend on the histology and staging of the lymphoma. However, modified chemotherapy regimes are usually necessary both to minimize toxicity in patients with limited bone marrow reserve due to their HIV infection and to reduce the risk of further drug-associated immuno-suppression. Less chemotherapy and the underlying immunosuppression diminish the likelihood of a complete response.

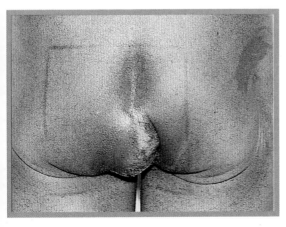

← 571 Non-Hodgkin's lymphoma of the rectum
The rectangular area shows the site for radiotherapy.

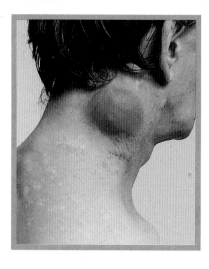

← 572 Non-Hodgkin's lymphoma in the neck
The patient was reasonably immunocompetent with a CD4 count of >400mm^3. He responded well to standard chemotherapy.

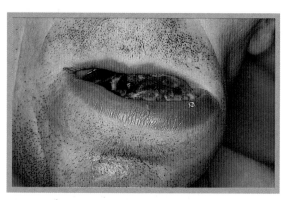

← 573 Non-Hodgkin's lymphoma in the mouth
Rapidly growing tumour in late stage HIV disease and poor prognosis.

Other malignancies

A number of other cancers occur more commonly in HIV disease ranging from **Hodgkin's lymphoma**, various **squamous cell carcinomas** and **testicular cancers**. Whether these are all truly increased in HIV disease or sometimes chance associations will require further case-controlled data. Notwithstanding, the clinical presentation and course of these rarer cancers is likely to be altered in the setting of HIV infection.

Cervical cancer and anal squamous cancer are discussed on page 257 in the section on interaction of HIV and sexually transmitted diseases (see **507**).

NEUROLOGICAL PRESENTATIONS

About 10% of initial AIDS-defining disease is due to neurological illness, with probably at least half of patients ultimately experiencing some neurological manifestations. Both the central and peripheral nervous system may be involved either due to a direct effect of HIV or as a consequence of immunosuppression. The resultant opportunistic infections and tumours are particularly likely to present as CNS mass lesions.

Intracranial mass lesions

Cerebral toxoplasmosis is the most common cause of a CNS space-occupying lesion in patients with AIDS, followed by **primary CNS lymphoma**, **progressive**

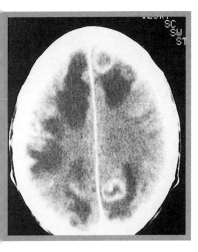

↑ **574 Toxoplasma brain abscesses**
Multiple ring-enhancing lesions are highly suggestive of Toxoplasma brain abscesses. This patient was treated empirically with pyrimethamine and sulphadiazine with good response. MRI scans are somewhat more sensitive and may show lesions earlier when the CT scan is negative.

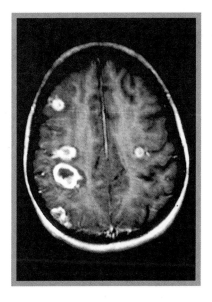

↑ **575 Cerebral toxoplasma**
Multiple thin-walled, ring-enhancing, toxoplasma lesions near the corticomedullary junctions in both parietal lobes. This is shown on an axial T1-weighted MRI following intravenous contrast enhancement.

multifocal leukoencephalopathy (PML) and other infectious agents, such as **candida**, *Mycobacterium tuberculosis* and **cryptococcus.** Focal signs may be present, which vary depending on the location of the mass. Diagnosis can be presumptively established in some cases by CT and MRI scanning. Brain biopsy should be considered where there is doubt and failure of empirical antitoxoplasma therapy.

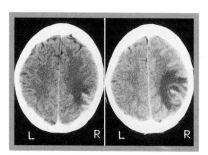

← **576 Cerebral toxoplasmosis**
The CT scan on the right shows a right parietal lobe lesion with contrast enhancement and surrounding white matter oedema and effacement of the adjacent cortical sulci. The scan on the left, following antitoxoplasma therapy for 2.5 weeks, shows a reduction in white matter oedema and less mass effect.

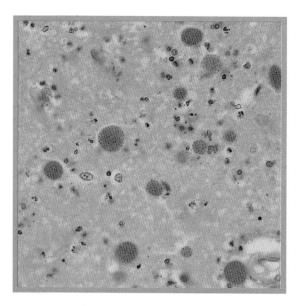

← **577 Cerebral toxoplasmosis**
Brain biopsy may be performed with atypical scans (see **576**) or if patients fail to respond to therapy for toxoplasmosis. This high-power section of brain shows numerous toxoplasma cysts.

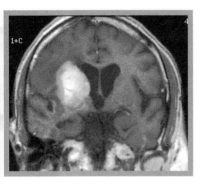

↑ **578 Cerebral high-grade B cell immunoblastic lymphoma (Epstein–Barr virus positive)**

Large right parietal, enhancing lymphomatous mass in a characteristic periventricular location. It is surrounded by low-signal oedema and is causing significant mass effect with effacement of the overlying cerebral sulci. This is shown in a coronal T1-weighted MRI following intravenous contrast enhancement.

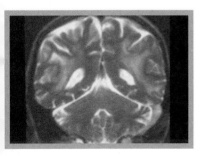

↑ **579 Progressive multifocal leukoencephalopathy (PML)**

This is a demyelinating disease of cerebral white matter. Bilateral parietal, high-signal lesions are shown on this coronal T2-weighted MRI scan. Note the sparing of the cortical grey matter and the absence of mass effect, which is characteristic of PML. Patients present with headache, ataxia, hemiparesis and confusion. Diagnosis is strongly suggested by typical MRI scans showing high-signal intensity lesions without enhancement. Cerebrospinal fluid (CSF) studies are usually unrevealing and diagnosis may be confirmed by polymerase chain reaction test for JC virus (a papovavirus) in the CSF.

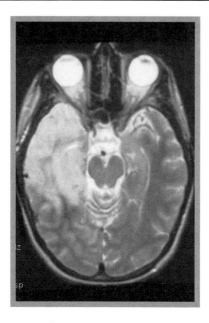

← 580 Herpes encephalitis
Swollen, high-signal, left temporal lobe cortical grey matter, characteristic in location and appearance of herpes encephalitis. Note the normal right temporal lobe for comparison in this axial T2-weighted MRI scan.

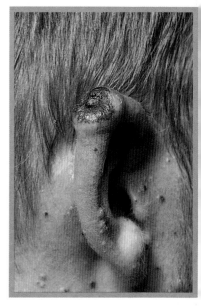

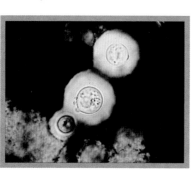

↑ 581 Cryptococcal meningitis in a patient with AIDS
The serum cryptococcal antigen test is usually positive. Examination of the cerebrospinal fluid may show these typical budding yeasts stained by Indian ink.

↑ 582 Disseminated cryptococcosis: skin lesions
Disseminated cryptococcosis may lead to skin lesions with a central umbilication resembling molluscum contagiosum. This patient also had meningism and the cryptococcal antigen titre was >1:400 000.

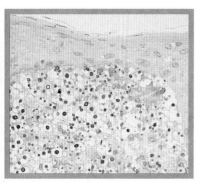

← 583 Disseminated cryptococcosis: skin lesions

Histology of skin lesions shown in **582**. High-power view of PAS strain showing intact epidermis overlying a mucoid-type infiltrate of the dermis composed of large numbers of cryptococci.

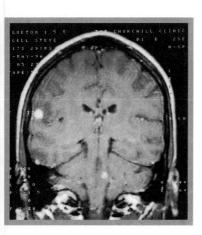

← 584 Multiple drug-resistant tuberculosis (MDRTB)

Postcontrast coronal T1-weighted MRI showing characteristic tuberculomata lesions. The patient had multiple drug-resistant TB (MDRTB) which was the reason for treatment failure and eventual dissemination.

HIV and the brain

The human immunodeficiency virus enters the CNS early and may cause **meningoencephalitis** or **inflammatory neuropathy** at the time of seroconversion illness (**527, 528**). It is unusual to find significant neurological impairment during the clinically latent stage of HIV disease, although there may be some abnormalities in the CSF including mononuclear pleocytosis, and slow wave EEG changes of uncertain significance.

Dementia

The term **HIV encephalopathy** is used to describe a progressive neurocognitive syndrome also known as **AIDS dementia complex (ADC)**. It is a late complication of HIV infection and the onset is usually insidious, with features such as loss of memory, poor concentration, lack of energy and depressive mood changes, although occasionally the patient may present as a psychiatric emergency with hypomania. The early signs of cognitive loss can be difficult to detect; as the illness progresses, the intellectual deterioration becomes more marked and often motor signs of ataxia and weakness appear. Neuropsychometric testing may be helpful and CT and MRI scans reveal a generalized atrophy that is (usually) inconsistent with the patient's age (**585, 586**).

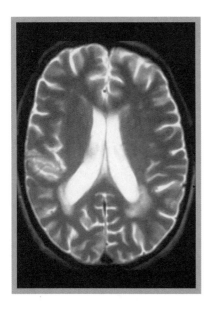

↑ 585 HIV encephalopathy
Diffuse cerebral atrophy with coarse periventricular white matter high signal, which is not extending out to the cortical grey matter, as is the case in the patient with progressive multifocal leukoencephalopathy (see **579**). Axial T2-weighted MRI scan.

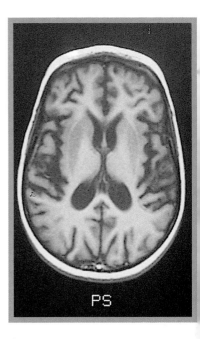

↑ 586 Marked generalized cerebral atrophy,
as shown in an axial T1-weighted MRI scan of a child with failure to thrive, spastic paraparesis and marked HIV dementia.

Peripheral neuropathies

The commonest pattern is of a gradual onset of painful sensory peripheral neuropathy in patients with advanced disease. The patients complain of increasingly painful dysaesthesia starting in the feet, which may lead to difficulty in walking and disturbed sleep. Differential diagnosis includes drug-induced neuropathy. Other manifestations, include inflammatory demyelinating polyneuropathies, either chronic or acute (Guillain–Barré syndrome). In addition, rarer neuropathies include mononeuritis multiplex and polyradiculopathy associated with cytomegalovirus infection.

OCULAR PRESENTATIONS

Cytomegalovirus (CMV) retinitis

This is a sight-threatening manifestation of HIV. It occurs in patients with profound immunodeficiency and CD4 counts are usually below 50/mm^3. Typically patients complain of blurred vision, 'floaters' and field defects. Untreated, this necrotizing retinitis can rapidly progress to irreversible blindness. Ophthalmological assessment and treatment is therefore urgent. Characteristic appearances are shown in **587**.

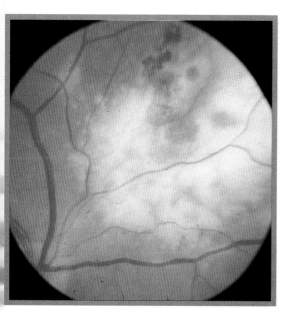

← 587 CMV retinitis
showing typical retinal infiltrates.

A number of other intraocular opportunistic infections have been recognised in patients with HIV and require expert ophthalmological management. They include **retinitis** due to **herpes simplex, herpes zoster (588)** and **Toxoplasma retinochoroiditis (589)** (with or without concurrent cerebral involvement). Other infections, seen very occasionally, are disseminated infections, such as those due to *Pneumocystis carinii* (590), *Cryptococcus neoformans, Treponema pallidum* and *Mycobacterium avium complex.*

Other HIV-related eye disease includes **HIV microvasculopathy** or 'cottonwool spots' which may be confused by the inexperienced with **cytomegalovirus (CMV).** They do not appear to be clinically significant (591).

External eye complaints are common and include blepharitis associated with seborrhoeic dermatitis and dry eyes, often as part of the **sicca syndrome.** Mucocutaneous viral infections, such as **molluscum contagiosum (505), herpes simplex** and **herpes zoster**, sometimes involve the external eye and cutaneous Kaposi's sarcoma may also affect the eyelids (**564**) and conjunctivae.

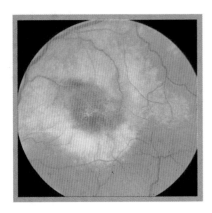

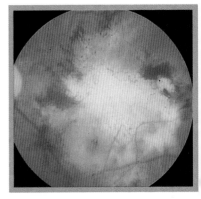

↑ 588 Progressive outer retinal necrosis (PORN)
usually associated with varicella zoster virus. This is usually rapidly progressive and leads to blindness.

↑ 589 Toxoplasma retinochoroiditis.

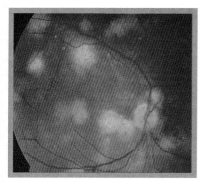

← 590 Disseminated PCP: choroidal lesions
(see also **545**).

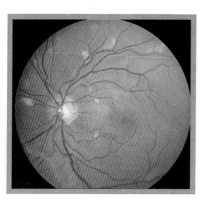

← 591 'Cottonwool spots'
are very commonly found in patients with HIV disease and AIDS, but have not been associated with the development of other retinal disease.

ALIMENTARY TRACT PRESENTATIONS

Patients with symptomatic HIV disease frequently present with gastrointestinal problems, most commonly due to secondary infection. Principal complaints include abdominal pain, weight loss, diarrhoea and perianal problems. There are often oral cavity and oesophageal symptoms.

Oral candidal involvement is common, appearing as erythematous or with pseudomembranous plaques (**592–594**). The oesophagus may be involved (occasionally without oral signs), leading to pain (**odynophagia**) and **dysphagia** (**595**). **Dental problems** may be florid, particularly **gingivitis**, which has led to patients presenting with severe **halitosis** (**596**). Dentists may also refer patients on seeing lesions of Kaposi's sarcoma involving the palate or gums (**561, 563**). **Oral hairy leukoplakia (OHL)**, which is caused by Epstein–Barr virus infection associated with HIV immunosuppression, produces characteristic corrugated lesions typically on the side of the tongue (**597**), but may also occur on the opposing buccal mucosa. Finally, **oral ulceration** may be severe and due either to specific infections with **herpes simplex** (**598**) or **cytomegalovirus,** or nonspecific **aphthous ulceration** (**595**). These latter three conditions may also cause dysphagia (**600**), although *Candida* remains the commonest cause. Diagnosis is by endoscopy and biopsy.

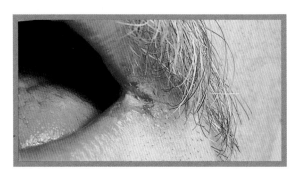

← **592 Angular cheilitis**
may be associated with oral candidiasis.

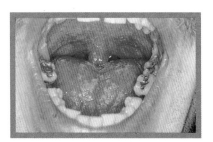

← **593 Erythematous candidiasis**
Note white plaques of candida on a diffuse erythematous background and oedema of the uvula. Oral candidiasis often occurs earlier in smokers.

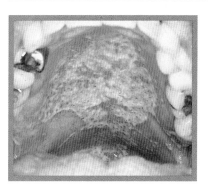

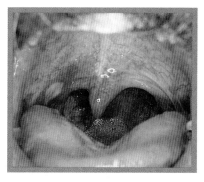

↑ **594 Pseudomembranous candidiasis**
Large plaque of oral thrush affecting hard palate.

↑ **595 Severe aphthous ulceration**
is a common complication in HIV. Lesions may also occur in the oesophagus and cause dysphagia.

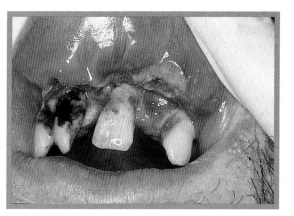

← **596 Severe necrotizing gingivitis**
The patient's initial presentation with HIV disease was halitosis.

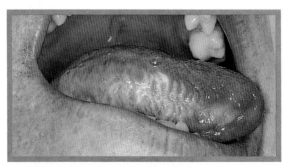

← 597 Typical ribbed appearance of oral hairy leukoplakia (OHL) on the side of the tongue.

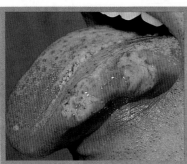

← 598 Oral herpes virus (HSV) may cause florid oral lesions such as these.

Abdominal pain may be due to tumours, such as lymphoma or KS involvement of the stomach (**601**), or due to specific infections, particularly CMV colitis (**602**). Diarrhoea is a common complaint and a specific cause can usually be found (**603**). Infective agents include traditional pathogens, such as **giardia**, **salmonella** and **shigella**, as well as opportunistic infection due **cryptosporidia**, **microsporidia**, and *Isospora belli* (**604–607**). Weight loss may be severe (**'slim disease'**) and associated with florid diarrhoea (**608**). However, acute opportunistic infection elsewhere may lead to weight loss. At late stages of disease, further weight loss is often due to inadequate intake rather than major malabsorption.

Cryptosporidia, microsporidia and CMV may also be associated with biliary tract disease and a condition called 'AIDS-related sclerosing cholangitis' (ARSC) (**609**). Patients present with severe upper quadrant pain and obstructive liver function tests. Hepatosplenomegaly is usually due to opportunistic infection, such as chronic hepatitis B, hepatitis C or mycobacterial infection.

Perianal pain is frequently due to recrudescence of **herpes simplex virus** (**500, 610**). **Perianal warts** may be florid (**506**).

An increase in **cloacogenic cell carcinoma** has been recorded (**507**).

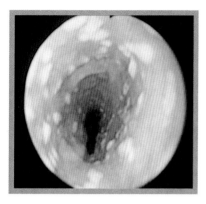

← 599 Oesophageal plaques of *Candida*
seen through the endoscope.

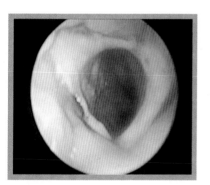

← 600 Cytomegalovirus (CMV) ulceration
proved to be an additional cause of this patient's dysphagia. The distal oesophageal ulceration is typical of cytomegalovirus. These endoscopic findings are from the same patient as in **599**.

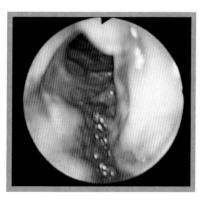

← 601 KS of the stomach
may be the cause of abdominal pain, seen here involving the pyloric canal.

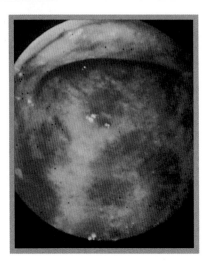

← 602 Cytomegalovirus colitis
viewed by endoscopy.

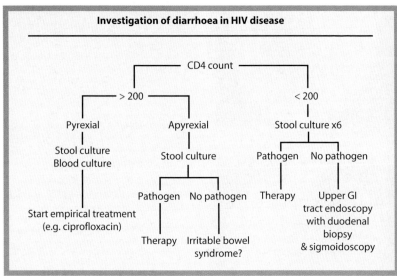

Investigation of diarrhoea in HIV disease

CD4 count
- > 200
  - Pyrexial
    - Stool culture
    - Blood culture
    - Start empirical treatment (e.g. ciprofloxacin)
  - Apyrexial
    - Stool culture
      - Pathogen → Therapy
      - No pathogen → Irritable bowel syndrome?
- < 200
  - Stool culture x6
    - Pathogen → Therapy
    - No pathogen → Upper GI tract endoscopy with duodenal biopsy & sigmoidoscopy

↑ 603 Algorithm showing the investigation of diarrhoea in HIV disease
The likelihood of 'pathogen-negative' diarrhoea in the <200 group decreases
with appropriate investigations.

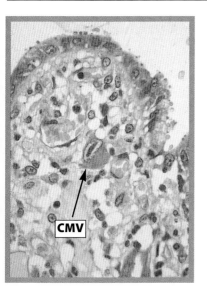

← 604 Concurrent infection with cryptosporidia and CMV infection

It is important to remember that dual infections are not uncommon. High-power view of small bowel villi showing numerous cryptosporidia adherent to the superficial enterocyte, and concurrent CMV infection with typical CMV inclusion cell in the lamina propria.

CMV

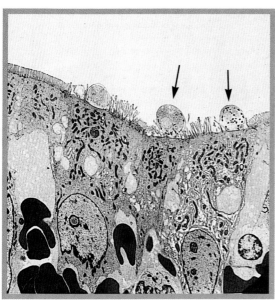

← 605 Cryptosporidia

Electron micrographs of cryptosporidia (arrowed) adherent to the microvillous surface of the enterocytes, with the associated loss of the normal microvillous structure.

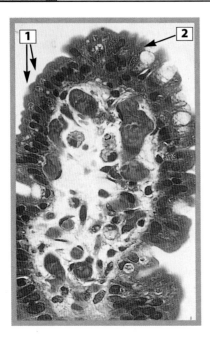

← 606 Microsporidia
High-power view of a small bowel villus showing numerous intracytoplasmic inclusions and small spores of microsporidia. **1:** mesont/sporont; **2:** spores (refractile).

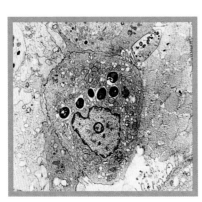

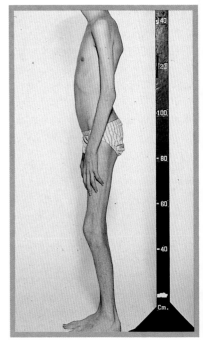

↑ 607 Microsporidia
Electron micrograph of enterocytes containing a number of dark-stained microsporidial spores.

↑ 608 'Slim' disease
HIV-associated wasting in a 19-year-old homosexual with severe cryptosporidial diarrhoea.

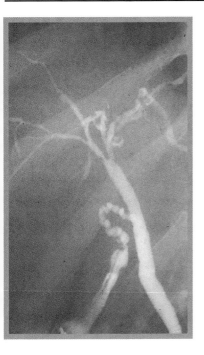

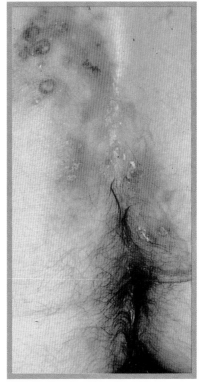

↑ 609 AIDS-related sclerosing cholangitis (ARSC)
Endoscopic retrograde cholangiopancreatographic (ERCP) opacification of the intrahepatic and extrahepatic biliary tree. The multiple intrahepatic strictures shown are characteristic of AIDS-related sclerosing cholangitis (ARSC).

↑ 610 Perianal herpes
Frequently recurrent or persistent lesions (without therapy) become more common with increasing immunosuppression.

SKIN DISEASE

The skin is a very sensitive indicator of immunosuppression and there is always some skin involvement in HIV disease. Cutaneous manifestations may be divided into infectious, non-infectious and malignant. Many examples of the first and last of these categories have already been illustrated and are cross-referenced.

Malignant disease

Lymphoma and **Kaposi's sarcoma** with its prominent skin involvement are discussed earlier (**556–573**). It has not been clearly determined whether other skin tumours, such as **malignant melanoma** or **non-melanoma skin cancers**, occur with increased frequency. They may, however, act more aggressively (**507**).

Infectious mucocutaneous manifestations in HIV

Fungal	Viral	Bacterial
Dermatophyte	HIV exanthema	Gram positive
Pityrosporum	Varicella zoster	e.g.*Staphylococus aureus*
Candida species	Herpes simplex	
Deep mycoses	Human papilloma	Gram negative
e.g.*Penicillium marneffei*	Molluscum contagiosum	e.g. *Pseudomonas aeruginosa*
Histoplasmosis		
Coccididomycosis		*Bartonella* species
Blastomycosis	Epstein–Barr	*B. henselae*
Aspergillosis	Cytomegalovirus	*B. quintana*
Sporotrichosis		
Zygomycosis	**Ectoparasites**	*Treponema* species
Pseudallercheria Boydii		*T. pallidum*
	Scabies	*T. pertenue*
		Mycobacteria
		MTB
		MAC
		Other mycobacteria
		Nocardiosis

↑ **611 Infectious mucocutaneous manifestations of HIV.**

Infectious cutaneous manifestations

A widened clinical spectrum of opportunistic infection on the skin is seen and a high level of clinical suspicion is necessary (**611**). Atypical manifestations are common and rare organisms sometimes seen. If in doubt, skin lesions should be biopsied (a 'punch' is usually sufficient) and a sample sent for histology and culture, preferably prior to any treatment.

Fungal infections

The high incidence of **seborrhoeic dermatitis** in HIV disease is probably related to increased populations of the likely causative organism, *Pityrosporum ovale* (**612, 613**). **Pityriasis versicolor** (**380**) and *Pityrosporum* **folliculitis** are also more common in seropositive individuals. **Dermatophyte infections**, particularly tinea pedis, is frequent and sometimes extensive, with additional nail involvement (**614, 615**).

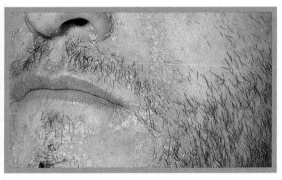

← 612 Severe seborrhoeic dermatitis

may be a presenting feature of HIV disease. Typical sites are the nasolabial folds, moustache and other hairy areas.

→ 613 Seborrhoeic dermatitis
may extend beyond its usual central sternal area.

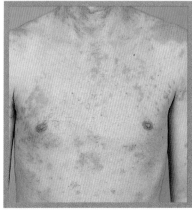

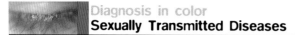
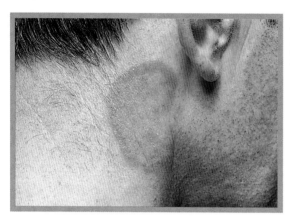

← 614
Dermatophyte infection
Tinea corporis.

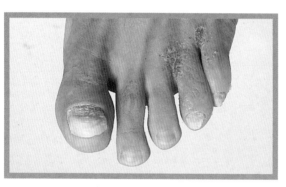

← 615
Dermatophyte infections
Dermatophytes may cause troublesome tinea pedis and onychomycosis as shown here.

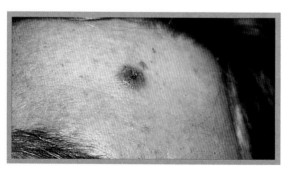

← 616
Disseminated histoplasmosis
Note umbilicated lesion mimicking molluscum contagiosum. Differential diagnosis includes *P. marneffei* infection and cryptococcosis.

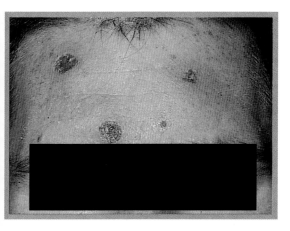

← 617
Blastomycosis hominis
Punched-out facial ulcers of *Blastomycosis hominis* in a patient who had lived in Southern Africa. Patient also had lung involvement with interstitial shadowing on the chest X-ray.

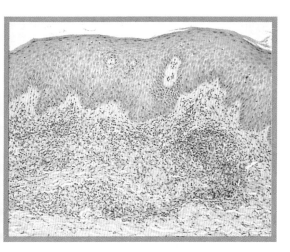

← 618
Blastomycosis hominis
Biopsy of trunk lesion from the same patient as shown in **617** showed granulomatous lesion and specific stain confirmed the diagnosis.

Disseminated infections with skin involvement are not uncommon, particularly in endemic areas. For example, ***Penicillium marneffei*** infection in the Far East, and **histoplasmosis** and **blastomycosis**, particularly in southern USA and South America. Skin biopsy, as suggested above, may aid diagnosis (**616-618**). **Cryptococcal** skin lesions are shown in **582**.

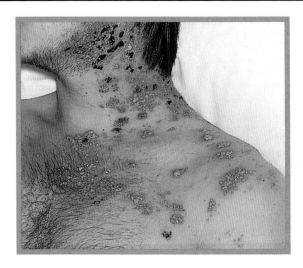

**← 619
Multidermatome
shingles**
is highly suggestive
of the immuno-
compromised state.

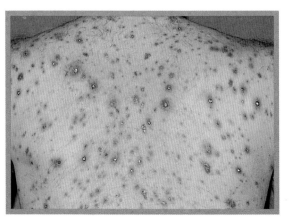

**← 620 Severe
disseminated
chickenpox**
may be seen in both
children and adults
in HIV disease.

Viral infections

The **rash** found in one-third of patients with primary HIV infection is described on pp. 275–277 (**527–531**).

Varicella zoster. This is often the first manifestation of HIV immunosuppression. **Herpes zoster** that covers three or more adjacent dermatomes, skips to discontinuous dermatomes or is accompanied by severe toxicity and disseminated chickenpox is particularly suggestive (**619, 620**). **Herpes simplex** which occurs with increasing frequency, severity or length of recurrences is found with progressive immunosuppression (**500, 501**). Less common forms include **disseminated herpes simplex infection (502, 503), chronic giant ulcerative herpes simplex** and **herpetic whitlow**, progressing to digital gangrene. Culture is usually sufficient, but occasionally biopsy from an atypical lesion is required to establish the diagnosis.

Human papillomavirus (HPV). Both genital and non-genital warts may be extensive, be more refractory to treatment and spread to unusual areas. Examples of genital warts are shown in (**506**) and the oncogenic potential should not be forgotten (**507**).

Molluscum contagiosum. These can be extensive or atypical, as described previously (**504, 505**). Giant forms are not uncommon. Umbilicated lesions may be simulated by deep fungal infections (**582, 616**).

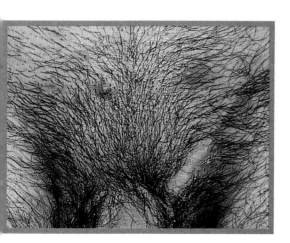

← 621 Staphylococcal folliculitis
This patient suffers from recurrent and often severe staphylococcal folliculitis.

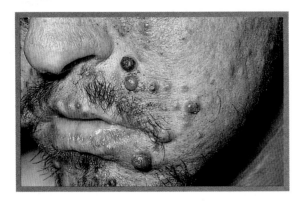

← 622 Bacillary angiomatosis (BA)
Striking cherry-like lesions of bacillary angiomatosis, with an appearance reminiscent of multiple pyogenic granulomata.

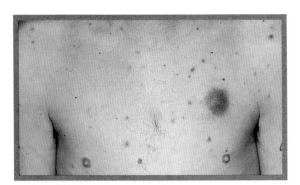

← 623 BA lesions on the chest
of the same patient as in **622**. Here, the lesions look more like Kaposi's sarcoma.

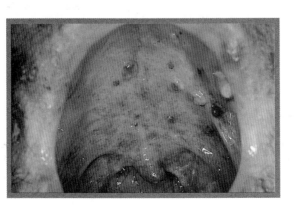

← 624 BA oral lesions
Oral lesions are sometimes seen with a similar, though smaller, cherry-like appearance. The patient also has warts of the palate.

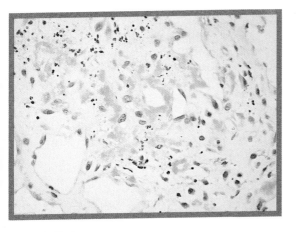

← 625 BA: high-power view (H&E stain), showing inflammation and angioproliferation with smudgy deposit in close association with the outer aspect of the capillary vasculature.

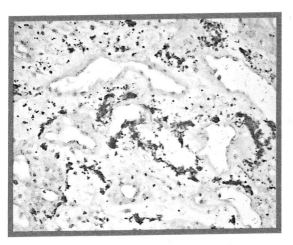

← 626 BA: high-power view (Warthin-Starry stain) The same case as in **625** with Warthin-Starry stain. The black-brown areas are compatible with the smudgy purplish areas in **625** indicative of positive staining for the bacteria.

Bacterial infections

Staphylococcus aureus is the most common cause of skin infection with folliculitis (**621**), impetigo, ecthyma or toxic scalded skin syndrome. Other organisms, such as *Pseudomonas aeruginosa* can cause ecthyma gangrenosum and panniculitis. A newly characterised bacterial infection is due to the *Bartonella* species, *Bartonella hensalae* or *B. quintana* (**622–626**). Involvement may spread to deeper tissues including the liver (**peliosis hepatitis**).

Mycobacterium tuberculosis. This microorganism may spread from underlying lymph nodes to the skin and **scrofuloderma (627)** can occur. Hypersensitivity reactions such as **papulonecrotic tuberculide** and **lupus vulgaris** are, in our experience, rare. At present, little is known about the interaction of HIV with *Mycobacterium leprae.* Bacterial sexually transmitted diseases, including syphilis in the context of HIV, have been described earlier (**508–510**).

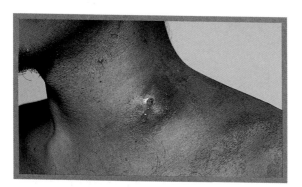

← 627
Scrofuloderma
Discharging tuberculous abscess. Note also molluscum contagiosum lesions on neck.

Infestations

Typical pruritic lesions may occur with **scabies** as in the seronegative (**444–451**). However, it is important to remember that itch is not a major feature of **crusted scabies (511–515)**, despite the massively increased number of mites.

Non-infectious manifestations
Pre-existing psoriasis
This may progress alarmingly and severe arthritis appears to be much more common (**628**).

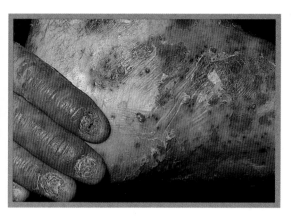

← 628 Psoriasis
may not occur more often in HIV disease, but will often be exacerbated, as in this patient.

Pruritus
This may be associated with very dry (**629**) or inflammatory conditions, such as **eosinophilic (itchy) folliculitis** (**630**). The latter is difficult to treat, although patients often improve with a holiday in the sun due to the ultraviolet light radiation. A variant involving the dermis is termed **pruritic papular eruption of HIV** and is said to be particularly troublesome in African patients.

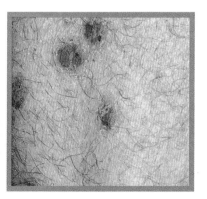

← 629 Dry skin
is often very troublesome and also pruritic. This patient has coexisting psoriasis.

325

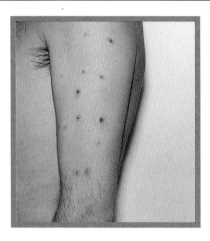

← 630 Eosinophilic 'itchy' folliculitis
Lesions are extremely pruritic and often number 50 or more. They may involve trunk and face, as well as limbs.

Allergic skin reactions to drugs
Allergic drug reactions appear to be much more frequent in HIV-infected patients. This may limit the use of antiretroviral therapies, or drugs used for treatment or prophylaxis against opportunistic infections. For example, some 30%–40% of patients are allergic to sulphur-containing drugs, such as cotrimoxazole which is used particularly against PCP. The likelihood of developing a rash with a particular agent appears to be related to the degree of immunosuppression in many cases. However, at a very late stage in the disease, the allergic potential seems to decrease again (**631, 632**).

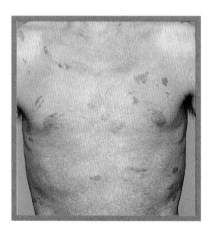

↑ 631 Allergic drug reactions
are common. Cotrimoxazole reaction in a patient who also has many Kaposi's sarcoma lesions.

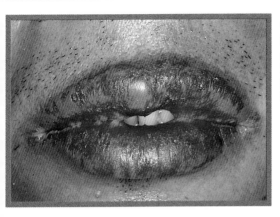

**↑632
Stevens–Johnson
syndrome**
Severe allergic reactions
may include mucosal
involvement.

HIV IN THE HAIR AND NAILS

Alopecia areata (**633**) is sometimes seen in common with other autoimmune diseases. Infection with HIV accelerates the ageing process and can induce **premature baldness**. **Hypertrichosis of the eyelashes** has been observed and so far has not been explained. **Nail involvement** includes **onychomycosis** (**615**), **candidal paronychia** and **nail psoriasis** (**628**).

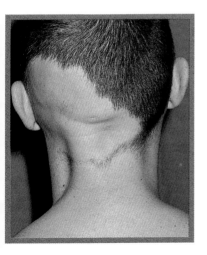

← 633 Alopecia areata
The frequency of alopecia areata is probably increased in HIV disease.

Index

A page number in normal type indicates a relevant illustration on that page; a page number in italic type indicates a relevant reference in text.

329

333